Transforming Social Work Practice

LI B

D1407081

TRANSFORMING SOCIAL WORK PRACTICE

Postmodern critical perspectives

Edited by Bob Pease and Jan Fook

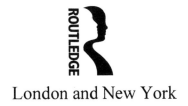

London and New York

First published in 1999 by Routledge
11 New Fetter Lane, London EC4P 4EE

Simultaneously published in the USA and Canada by Routledge
29 West 35th Street, New York, NY 10001

Set in 10/11 pt Sabon by DOCUPRO, Sydney
Printed by KHL Printing, Singapore

British Library Cataloging in Publication Data
A catalogue record for this book is available from the British Library

Library of Congress Cataloging in Publication Data
A catalogue record for this book has been requested

ISBN 0-415-21646-X (hb)
ISBN 0-415-21647-8 (pb)

Foreword

When, in 1848, Marx and Engels wrote in *The Communist Manifesto* their account of the processes of social transformation through which the dynamic development of capitalism was manifested, they spoke of dramatic changes which shook the very foundations of beliefs, customs and ways of living. They identified the cultural shock produced by these changes as being the 'uninterrupted disturbance of all social conditions', a succession of material and emotional crises which were experienced as 'everlasting uncertainty and agitation'. Marx and Engels were referring to what we would now call early capitalism, and we might compare the social revolution that they described to the everlasting uncertainty of the present: the late capitalism of a global economy accompanied by a growing culture of postmodern scepticism. Just as rapid and accelerating economic and social changes in the earlier stages of capitalism resulted in new approaches to the social management of the disorganisation, impoverishment and alienation of the casualties of 'progress'—upon which social work was founded—the profound changes that are now taking place in economies, cultures and identities are having their stunning impact on the ideas and practices of contemporary social work across the world. It is to this impact that *Transforming Social Work Practice: Postmodern Critical Perspectives* is a response, one which reaches out from the critical tradition in social work to interrogate postmodernism's own critique and incorporate it, where possible, into a radical emancipatory social work theory and practice.

In order to pursue the project of a reconstructed critical social work practice, it is necessary to recognise the profound challenge with which postmodernism confronts the paradigms of critical social work itself. We might speak of these unsettling times in terms of dramatic shifts in international economic conditions directed to increasing the rate of exploitation of people and nature, and point with apprehension to the media-led manufacture of desire. What is perhaps most significant for critical social work at this juncture, however, is the postmodern challenge that is being mounted to the foundational beliefs upon which Western societies gradually developed both their social institutions and their conceptions of the individual person over the past two hundred years. Many of these beliefs—in fundamental human rights, the relative autonomy of the individual subject, the notion of social progress through the application of reason—have formed the basis of the revolutionary and critical tradition, within Western culture, which has struggled against class, gender and colonial oppression in the name of universal values. All of these beliefs are now treated with profound scepticism and suspicion, if not outright hostility, by many postmodern critics.

As the postmodern evaluation of modernity proceeds, it becomes, I believe, increasingly convincing as a challenge to the arrogance, the hubris, of Western claims to universal knowledge rooted in a linear idea of scientific and social progress. These claims have led to deeply flawed projects of emancipation, one version of which was inaugurated by Marx and very nearly, but not quite, destroyed by Stalin. What we must now face is the recognition that the critical tradition, of which one stream of social work practice is part, was itself implicated in varying degrees with a Western triumphalism which, in its turn, legitimated economic exploitation, women's subordination, neo-colonialism, homophobia, racism and other oppressions. The knowledge claims of modernity, based on a dogmatic belief in one universal Truth, have been instrumental in silencing, erasing or marginalising the diverse voices, needs and practices of the Other.

So the question becomes this: How can we maintain what was positive and liberating in the critical tradition in social work, the emancipatory side of the Enlightenment, but still use postmodernism to deconstruct the problematic elements in the metanarratives of feminism, Marxism, and other critical perspectives to the point where reconstruction becomes possible? *Transforming Social Work Practice* contributes a range of theoretical and practice answers to this question in a way which is exceptionally stimulating and provocative. Its approach involves a continuous challenge to categories established under the regime of universal Truth: the exclusive and hierarchically placed opposites of male/female, heterosexual/homosexual, theory/practice, expert/client, teacher/taught, true/false. This deconstructive approach enables the contributors to re-examine the connection between social work theorisation and the actual practices of social workers. A number of the chapters draw directly or indirectly on the narratives of those predominantly seen as 'outside of theory', front-line practitioners and service users who in most professional discourses on theory are not authorised to speak. But to open the discourse on a reconstructed critical social work practice to previously excluded voices requires, the book argues, a re-examination of the concepts of power and resistance, the assertion of the continuous possibility of individuals acting as moral agents within specific structural pre-conditions, and a strong commitment to the acknowledgment and celebration of difference.

Many of the writers in this book, including the editors, Bob Pease and Jan Fook, could be classified within the division of social work labour as academics. We academics, this book demonstrates, are in a position to assist in the building, together with students and social work practitioners, of new and transformative kinds of knowledge, provided we can conceive of our educational and research practices as dialogical ones. If students, social workers and social work educators can see knowledge as culturally constructed, then together we can engage in the deconstruction of received ideas by revealing their discursive contradictions and consequently test the extent to which dominant narratives can unwittingly provide the spaces for transgression and resistance.

I found while reading this book that I was frequently provoked to engage in critical reflection on my own teaching and writing. I recall, as I write this Foreword, a graduate seminar on the social construction of subjectivity which I have taught for several years. At one meeting of this seminar, we had, as is often the case, come to the painful but barely tolerable realisation that none of us could avoid being implicated in discourses and practices of domination and exclusion. As we explored, in this particular instance, how we were socially constructed by the racism and homophobia profoundly internalised within our subjectivities, rage and guilt flowed amongst us. I searched for a way to escape the sheer emotional intensity of what the seminar was releasing. I chose the characteristic academic path of intellectual defence, the escape to *theorising* about racism and homophobia, a path which the seminar participants found themselves eager to follow. Racism and homophobia could be displaced from the immediate interactions amongst us, the product of our moral agency located within our socially constructed subject positions, and instead be located 'out there' in the exercise of oppressive institutional power far removed from the room in which we were sitting. Later, when we trusted each other more, we were able to acknowledge that the escape to theorisation, instigated by me, the teacher, was in this instance a denial of our everyday experience of the diffusion of power, of the multiple and complex nature of oppression, and of the problematics of living as if each of us had only one fixed identity rather than multiple and contradictory subjectivities. The postmodern style of reflection, the attempt to let go of the comforts of familiar metanarratives, enabled us eventually to begin the process of deconstructing our educational practices in the seminar and learn something about the contradictions we often experience in the dialectic of theory and practice.

This book is, I believe, a powerful intervention in the debate about the uncertain future of all kinds of social work, including that which continues within a critical tradition. Its power comes from the editors' and contributors' determination to question the ideas of the critical tradition of which they are part, and to transgress the exclusive binary category of theory/practice, showing us how the theories can emerge from the practices of the local and of the resistant Other. This is a book which deserves to be read and debated by social workers, students and social work educators in the many countries where the function of welfare and the role of social work is being subjected to intense scrutiny. In a world of multinational corporations intent on escalating the exploitation of the most disadvantaged and impoverished of populations, we must ask ourselves how human welfare can anywhere, even in the West, be defended and enhanced. *Transforming Social Work Practice: Postmodern Critical Perspectives* is a significant contribution to one part of this wider question: What is to be done about social work in 'advanced' capitalist countries and how might we begin to provide necessarily provisional answers?

Peter Leonard
McGill University, Montreal

Contents

Contributors

Lister Bainbridge is a Senior Lecturer in Social Work and Community Welfare at James Cook University of North Queensland.

Linda Briskman is a Senior Lecturer in Social Work at Deakin University.

Peter Camilleri is Associate Professor of Social Work at the Australian Catholic University in Canberra. He is author of *Reconstructing Social Work* (Avebury).

Karen Crinall currently lectures in Social Welfare at Monash University, Gippsland.

Lee FitzRoy lectures in Social Work at RMIT University, Melbourne.

Jan Fook is currently Professor of Social Work at Deakin University in Geelong, whilst on secondment from La Trobe University. She is the author of *Radical Casework* (Allen & Unwin) and editor of *The Reflective Practitioner* (Allen & Unwin).

Karen Healy is a Lecturer in the Department of Social Work, Social Policy and Sociology at the University of Sydney.

Gary Hough is a Senior Lecturer in Social Work at RMIT University, Melbourne.

Jim Ife is Professor of Social Work and Social Administration at the University of Western Australia. He is author of *Community Development: Creating Community Alternatives—Vision, Analysis and Practice* (Longman) and *Rethinking Social Work: Towards Critical Practice* (Longman).

Helen Jessop has worked as a teacher, practitioner and manager in the social work field and is currently based in Tasmania.

Mary Lane is a Senior Lecturer in the Department of Social Work, Social Policy and Sociology at the University of Sydney.

Carolyn Noble is a Senior Lecturer in Social Work at the University of Western Sydney.

Steve Parker is a social worker at Hanover Welfare Services in Melbourne.

Bob Pease is a Senior Lecturer in Social Work at RMIT University, Melbourne. He is the author of *Men and Sexual Politics: Towards a Profeminist Practice* (Dulwich).

Steve Rogerson is currently working in social welfare education and practice in Tasmania.

1 Postmodern critical theory and emancipatory social work practice
Bob Pease and Jan Fook

What does postmodern critical theory offer in shaping directions for social work practice? This is the question that motivated us to bring together this collection of papers.

The book grew out of a series of lunchtime discussions in 1995 and 1996 between social work academics in Melbourne who were interested in discussing the implications of postmodernism for progressive practice in social work. At that time, there was little social work literature on the development of postmodern social theory and there was even less engagement with postmodernism by radical social work writers.

The book is thus a collaborative attempt to define and develop a new discourse of theory and practice in social work which we call postmodern critical social work.[1] A specific focus of this book is bringing together contemporary theoretical and empirical work by a range of social work researchers who are involved in working through the implications of postmodern critical theory for social work practice. Most of the contributors to this volume are involved in attempts to construct emancipatory approaches to practice in specific fields of social work. The book is thus a contribution to the wider struggle of deconstructing traditional social work in order to formulate strategies of emancipatory practice.

In this introductory chapter, we provide some personal and theoretical background to the development of emancipatory perspectives in social work. We then locate the book within the context of the current theoretical debates about postmodernism and consider their implications for the future of emancipatory social work. The last section summarises our version of postmodern critical theory and shows how the various chapters address this perspective.

WHY THE POSTMODERN TURN? BOB'S STORY

I felt a strong sense of disquiet during my education as a social worker. I had an intuitive reaction against much of what was taught under the rubric of social work theory and practice. I had no systematic political analysis at this time and I suspect that some of my rebellion stemmed from my own lived experience of working-class life, as much of this was at odds with the middle-class conceptions of working-class clients conveyed to students in the classroom.

The integration of theory and practice was of particular interest to me and I struggled hard to relate the theoretical and technical knowledge of the classroom to the realities of my placement experiences. Although there were educational expectations that these should be integrated, little guidance was provided on how one actually did this.

With six months to go before graduating, I decided to take a year's leave of absence from social work to examine these issues more thoroughly. During this time, I studied political economy and became involved in activist community politics. I became clearer about my own purposes and about what theories I wanted to integrate with what practices.

At this time, I came to see the relevance of a Marxist analysis for understanding many of the issues that social workers were confronted with. But I had little understanding of how one could utilise this framework in daily practice. I had grasped some Marxist insights about the social world, but I had no understanding of the dialectical method that Marx used to derive these insights and hence no way to use such a method to construct a radical practice. During this time, I began to feel the impact of the women's movement and feminist analyses, so I began to temper my developing Marxist analysis with a feminist understanding of personal–political connections. These connections were further affirmed through the influence of the radical therapy movement. In addition to these theoretical influences, I gained my first apprenticeship as a community organiser in the fields of housing, unemployment and health issues.

With a clearer sense of social purpose and a political practice behind me, I returned to the study of social work and finished my degree. Upon graduation, I obtained a job as a community development officer in the 'dying days' of the Australian Assistance Plan (AAP). Following the demise of the AAP, I coordinated a resource centre for community action groups. Much of my work during this time involved the establishment of alternative community-based social services projects. In the development of these services, we endeavoured to create alternative collectivist/demo-cratic structures and aimed to link service provision with collective action. In this context I began to explore the implications of class and gender analyses for direct service work. At about this time, there were early attempts to construct paradigms for radical practice (Galper 1975; Bailey and Brake 1975; Corrigan and Leonard 1978). Being located outside the state maximised oppor-tunities for these radical frameworks to be tested out in practice.

Throughout the time I was associated with these alternative social services, I monitored and assessed my attempts to relate the radical models to my practice. To facilitate this self-evaluation of practice, I set up a study/support group of progressive social workers, maintained a daily diary of my work and wrote a series of discussion papers on my practice. I did not conceptualise these activities at the time as research. They were just my attempts to make sense of what I was doing. It has taken me a long time to validate this reflective practice as research and to recognise the potential within such research for the generation of new knowl-edge.

At the time, however, I thought that theorising and teaching in academia would provide opportunities for exploring the many unanswered questions that my practice and my reflections upon it had raised. So I entered social work education in 1980. In the practice subjects that I taught, I was able to bring together some of my practice and experience with my developing structural analysis. But, of course, I did not have all the answers and the available radical social work literature left much to be desired, as I knew from my own practice.

I felt a need for my own theorising to be more grounded in the practice reality of social workers. I thus began a collaborative inquiry into the attempts of radical practitioners to construct progressive practices in their work (Pease 1987, 1990). In the early days of this research, I hoped to construct a model of radical practice by integrating the experiences of the practitioners into a coherent practice framework. What I found, however, was a plurality of radical approaches. During the research, a multiplicity of views were expressed about both radical analysis and strategy in social work. Rather than try to encapsulate them within a framework of my own making, I constructed a one-act play to allow the different voices to be heard. At this point, I had never heard of postmodernism; looking back now, however, I realise that this was my first step towards a postmodern theorising about political practice.

It would be some years later when I enrolled in a doctorate to theorise the subjectivities and practices of profeminist men that

I would revisit these questions (Pease 1996). From my first encounters with feminist literature in the 1970s, I had been influenced by feminist theorising about men. However, this did not provide specific guidance for practice because the subject of men has not been given a central priority in feminist theorising. I had explored sex role theory and psychoanalytical and Jungian ideas, but I soon came to recognise the limitations of these theories for examining men's social power and institutionalised dominance. I then examined social constructionist approaches to masculinity that emphasised men's material and economic position and their social practices at home and at work. In the end, I found these approaches limiting as well because they did not provide sufficient guidance on how men could change their subjectivities and practices. I thus found myself confronting the same dilemmas I had encountered when practising, teaching and researching radical social work. To work through these issues, I began to read about the intersections of feminism, postmodernism and critical theory and to consider the implications these developments had for changing men and masculinities.

As I report in detail in Chapter 7, postmodern critical theory enabled me to move beyond the dualism that existed between voluntarism and structural determinism. I began to see how non-patriarchal subject positions for men could be discursively produced and how it was possible for men to reformulate their interests to challenge gender domination. It gave me a sense of agency in the face of the material and social basis of patriarchy. It also provided a language with which to revisit the unresolved dilemmas I had encountered with structural approaches to social work practice (Moreau 1990; Mullaly 1993), the more contemporary expressions of radical social work. The conversations that began to take place with Jan and other colleagues about these issues in 1995 became the basis for this book.

WHY THE POSTMODERN TURN? JAN'S STORY

As a young social worker in the late 1970s, I graduated with an awareness that casework was seen as inherently conservative, and that community work was seen as the 'right-minded' path to follow. Yet this simple dichotomy did not seem to me to fit the world of my early practice. I worked with people in my first job who, although strong and empowered volunteers—some of them trailblazers in the field of intellectual disability services—still needed emotional support, and sometimes more explicit counselling, to help them cope with the daily stresses of parenting children with intellectual disabilities.

My disquiet with this over-simplistic dichotomy, this forced choice of 'casework versus community work', carried over into my experience of postgraduate study, when I decided I would try to research the problem of 'radical casework'. What I found was another disquieting dichotomy, a world in which it seemed that male academic theorising sociologists tried to teach female practising social workers better social work by 'converting' them to a world of theory (e.g. Althusser), which incidentally seemed to be 'owned' by the male academic sociologists. Since I was neither male nor a sociologist, but was at the time an academic and a social worker, I found the dichotomy inadequate as a representation of my own experience and identity.

I had always had a love of theory, but did not feel that it had to come at the expense of practice. Neither could I see why community work had to be practised in the annihilation of casework, and similarly, I could not see why academic (and by definition, male) teaching had to necessarily devalue the experience of female practitioners. These were the beginnings of my disaffection with the culture of radicalism, although I was—and still am—a strong proponent of radical (and structural) social work analysis, I began to question many of the practical expressions, the lived experience, of radicalism.

I continued to observe instances in which the culture of radicalism seemed to me to be limited. For instance, in my teaching of radical casework practice, I am often struck by how students seem to think that 'radical' and 'traditional' practices must be, by definition, mutually exclusive. Therefore they feel they cannot use a skill radically if it has already been taught to them in a 'traditional' practice class. This type of thinking leads mostly to radical *in*action.

This phenomenon is similar to what I term a 'commodification' of theory, as if radical theory consists of a material set of ideas which can be transferred from one person to another. A person becomes radical if they can take on all the right ideas—they have thus become converted. This way of thinking, however, is potentially disempowering, since it assumes that the source of radicalism comes from 'outside' the person, and lies solely in the the acceptance of certain beliefs. There is a danger that the experience of the 'unconverted' will be devalued and discounted, and there is therefore potential for radicalism to be experienced as disempowering (by those who by definition don't have it).

Another example of how radicalism can be experienced as disempowering was put to me by one of my own students recently.

She related how, as a woman of South Asian heritage and appearance, she had felt quite disempowered when she came out of a class on structural social work which had clearly labelled people like herself as 'disadvantaged' and 'oppressed'. She hadn't felt that way before she went into the class, but she now felt that the source and cause of her 'problems' were located in the social structure (and so, by definition, the actions to address them must be too). She experienced a sense of classic alienation—a distancing from the ability to change her situation—because she had been labelled and categorised in a deterministic way.

For me, this potentially deterministic thinking also fails to account for my own experience in relation to another important aspect of my life. I happen to be of third-generation Australian-born Chinese descent. I appear racially Chinese, but have been raised with a primarily white Australian identity (as happened to many non-Anglo people during the 1950s in Australia). I do, in this sense, have one foot each in both the advantaged and disadvantaged classes. Simple structural analysis fails to be meaningful for my identity, because it fails to allow for seeming contradictions in people's behaviour and identities. These types of reflections on the limitations of theorising inherent in radicalism led me to examine much more closely the epistemological assumptions inherent in my own thinking.

At about the same time that I was becoming unhappy about the cultural expressions of social work radicalism, I became involved in developing a new postgraduate social work practice program. I realised, to my consternation, that I could not peddle the usual material (update on practice theories), since a good number of the potential students had only recently completed their undergraduate study (taught by me), and I could hardly teach them the same material again. I thus began to question why I even thought I should each them this type of material. What made me the expert, when it was *they* who were experiencing, and practising in, the current workplace? Having thus deconstructed my own position of authority rather neatly, I was still left in limbo without anything to teach (to students who would, alas, be paying higher fees and would expect more for their money). Fortunately, I was introduced to the reflective work of Argyris and Schon (1976).

It was in the thinking of the reflective approach, which questions the technological and rational approach to professional theory-building, that I found the connections with my own queries about the disempowering effects of radical thinking, which tends to devalue the lived experience of ordinary people. Instead of sets of ideas (invented by an expert) to which I must pay exclusive homage, and which are tested by their applicability, theories started becoming for me ways in which I could construct meaning and interpret my world in order to act within it. In this way of thinking, *I* drive the theory, rather than being theory-driven. The purpose of my classes thus became to assist students to build their own practice theory, directly from their own practice, through a process of reflection.

At the same time, I was acutely conscious, when facilitating class discussion, that I was guiding students to reflect upon structural and gender-related factors in their practice, often focusing on questions of power (this latter tended to be an issue raised spontaneously by students thememlves), and how these issues related to their own subjective positions and vice versa. I deliberately broadened the focus of reflection, so that our discussions could produce insights about how students could connect their personal experience and skills with strategies for acting in their work environments. I did not feel it was enough to simply be able to reflect upon, and build up, one's own theory—this occurs necessarily in a social, economic and cultural context, and must always be developed in relation to, and in interaction with, prevailing conditions. In this sense, then, I was implicitly working on a set of assumptions which acknowledged the structural world, but which focused on the ways in which we construct it through a process of interaction and dialogue. For me, this was the beginning of an engagement with more explicitly critical and postmodern and poststructural thinking. In Chapter 13, I outline the critical reflective approach and its relationship to critical postmodern thinking.

At this point in time, therefore, I subscribe to principles of radical practice in that I believe the mission of contemporary social work should be emancipatory. However, what I question are the implicit ways of thinking in radicalism which are disempowering. Therefore, for me, radical practice must be informed by postmodern cautions—it is not so much about matching radical practice strategies with radical theories, but undertaking a process of engaging with problem situations in order to change them along more emancipatory lines.

EMANCIPATORY PERSPECTIVES IN SOCIAL WORK: THE DEVELOPMENT OF CURRENT TRENDS

Having outlined our own personal pathways, it is relevant now to turn to social work literature more broadly. What trends are reflected in social work theorising about emancipatory practice over the last few decades?

Radical and structural social work

It is commonly agreed that emancipatory social work began with the development of radical critiques in the 1970s with British writers such as Bailey and Brake (1975, 1980), Corrigan and Leonard (1978), Galper (1975, 1980) in the United States and Throssell (1975) in Australia. In Canada, Maurice Moreau (1979) is generally credited with the initial naming of the structural approach, although this has most extensively been developed more recently by another Canadian, Bob Mullaly (1993, 1998). Besides their criticism of traditional social work as a victim-blaming and status quo-preserving enterprise, these approaches also had in common the imperative to focus on structural determinants of personal problems, and an inherent exhortation to personal liberaton and social change (Fook 1993; Payne 1997)—that is, an activist element (Healy, K. 1995).

Feminist social work

In the 1980s, radical and structural models were rightfully criticised for their lack of attention to gender dimensions, and feminist social work (Brook and Davis 1985; Marchant and Wearing 1986; Dominelli and Mcleod 1989) was developed more fully. Feminist social work models, in particular, were much better at developing the links between analysis and practice, and between personal and political experience—both dimensions which were largely ignored (or poorly developed) in earlier radical formulations. Indeed, a major current criticism of structural approaches to social work practice is the relative inattention given to the clinical, individual and interpersonal realms of practice (Cohen 1975). Although there has been a slight resurgence of writing from a radical social work perspective (e.g. Langan and Lee 1989; De Maria 1993; Thompson 1993) in the 1990s, it is still probably fair to say that the more personalised side of experience—and hence related models of practice—is still relatively underdeveloped.

Additionally, the structural, radical and feminist models of social work practice developed to date are mostly based on the principle that the aim of social work should be to empower less powerful people or groups. This, of course, assumes that the possession of power acts as the great divide in our social organisation, and that people generally either belong mutually exclusively to one of two groups: powerful or powerless, advantaged or disadvantaged, oppressor or oppressed, exploiter or exploited. The division usually occurs along gender, class, cultural or racial lines.

More recently, the trend has been to acknowledge the oversimplicity of such a binary analysis, and to turn to postmodern and poststructural formulations as a basis for understanding the complexities, contradictions and uncertainties of the contemporary world. In social work, this has taken several different forms.

Critical social science

Some writers have tried to re-emphasise the critical social science underpinnings of emancipatory social work (Ife 1996). Although acknowledging that postmodern or poststructural thinking shares some commonalities with a critical tradition, they are particularly dismayed by what they see as an overriding relativist tendency, which they argue is contradictory to the universalist truth claims inherent in a critical aproach (Piele and McCouat 1997). Postmodernism and poststructuralism are therefore rejected as adequate perspectives for pursuing the emancipatory social work project, and critical theory is reaffirmed as the fundamental guiding framework.

Postmodern and poststructural social work

There is, however, a growing body of literature which has come to use postmodernism or poststructuralism, or aspects of such thinking, in a number of different ways, to both analyse and develop emancipatory forms of social work practice. (For the purposes of this chapter—and indeed in this book generally—we make little distinction between postmodernism and poststructuralism. Although a distinction can be made (Healy and Fook 1994), we believe it is not significant enough to have a meaningful impact on the ideas in this book.)

In the United States, the debate about postmodernism and poststructuralism has primarily been played out through debates about research paradigms: constructivist/interpretivist versus positivist (Haworth 1991). Constructivism, or social constructionism, emphasises the ways in which individuals shape their world through ways of knowing and thinking, and thus shares elements with the poststructuralist idea of deconstructive or discursive analysis. Family therapists such as Hartmann (1990, 1991, 1992) and Laird (1993) have to some degree been interested in postmodernism, possibly because of its potential to deconstruct patterns of family functioning.

The work of Australian family therapist Michael White (White and Epston 1989; White 1995), based on explicit postmodern thinking, has become internationally recognised, and has been instrumental in propogating the usefulness of postmodern analysis in many types of clinical practice. Narrative analysis and techniques (Solas 1996; Parry and Doan 1994; Burman et al. 1996) are, of course, now widely used in both research and therapeutic settings. The acknowledgment of the new epistemological paradigms inherent in postmodern thinking has also meant that questions have arisen about all fields of social work endeavour. In this sense, the shift to postmodern thinking has meant that the traditional boundaries and relationships between theory, practice and research in social work have been reworked and redefined. While some literature has focused on affirming new ways of approaching research, and conceptualising practice in relation to research (e.g. Fook 1996; Ristock and Pennell 1996), other studies have focused on traditional ways of conceptualising the relatonships between theory and practice (Camilleri 1996; Harre Hindmarsh 1992), showing how such views have been problematic in the practice and education of social workers.

One of the earliest works to appear was Rojek et al. (1988), which consisted primarily of a deconstruction of the major forms of social work theorising to date. Later works noted the postmodern age in which social work was operating, particularly the influences of globalisation and the death of the welfare state (Parton 1994, 1996). These writers tried to map a future for welfare generally, and social work as a profession within it. Forecasts were varying in their optimism, but most argued strongly for the need for social work to transform itself from a traditional profession with a unified theory and practice base, and to learn to operate in diverse settings, with diverse value systems and population groups.

Some writers focused particularly on social work education, and attempted to deconstruct our present endeavours (Solas 1996) or point to ways in which poststructuralism changes social work education (Irwin et al. 1994; Leonard 1994; Featherstone and Fawcett 1995). A small body of literature looks specifically at the implications of postmodernism for social work practice (Pardeck et al. 1994; Healy and Fook 1994).

Postmodern critical theory

More recently, in acknowledgment that purely postmodern analysis does not necessarily provide guidelines—or even a moral basis—for responsible action, there have been more works which have tried to map out the connections between poststructuralism and critical social work (Rossiter 1996; Leonard 1997). This is the tradition into which this book fits. In the next section, we outline the features of a postmodern critical approach to social work, and show how specific chapters of the book address aspects of this analysis.

POSTMODERN CRITICAL THEORY AND SOCIAL WORK

The purpose of this section of the chapter is not to engage in broad theoretical discussions about key debates in postmodernism. Rather, we want to examine some of the main concepts that we think are useful for emancipatory approaches to social work and consider their implications for practice.

First, what is postmodernism? In its broadest sense, postmodernism involves a critique of all totalising theories—that is, theories which set out to explain everything (Tilley 1990: 327). It is said that the most compelling argument against totalising theories is that they give a one-sided, reductive perspective on social reality and so preclude the possibility of more multi-dimensional approaches (Kellner 1989: 177). To claim to speak for the universal is seen to deny the multifarious oppressions. Thus postmodernists believe that there is no one system of domination that holds pre-eminence over others.

What are the implications of this premise for social work? The dominant view in mainstream social work is that objective truth exists and can be discovered by value-free research. (See, for example, Grinnell 1988.) From a postmodern perspective, social workers do not have a monopoly on the truth. So we would reject those theories that posit an objective view of reality and would develop a critical attitude to all received ideas (Leonard 1994: 18).

A postmodern perspective also means that one needs to value uncertainty and to cultivate a modesty about one's political beliefs. Social workers would not attempt to define the experience of another group. As social workers, we should question how our cultural experience might cause us to privilege some aspects of reality and marginalise and disqualify others. We would encourage clients to collaborate in the construction of meaning associated with their experience (Pozatek 1994: 399).

In this view, there are no privileged positions. Meaning is constructed through conversation and dialogue. This requires social workers to allow their professional knowledge to be challenged (Hartman 1992: 484). We must reconsider the notion that social work is a unitary activity based on a coherent body of knowledge and expertise (Smith and White 1997: 283). We must also reject the idea that scientific imperatives and value-free techniques can be applied to individual and social problems (Irving 1994: 32).

Because of its acknowledgment of multiple realities, postmodernism is often criticised for drawing attention away from notions of social justice and common experiences of oppression (Taylor-Gooby 1994) and for lacking a coherent political program (Rossiter 1996: 29). The chapter by Jim Ife in this volume specifically addresses these criticisms. However, there are many forms of postmodernism reflecting the extent to which they break with notions of modernity and the extent to which they retreat from an emancipatory politics. These distinctions have been variously articulated as 'weak' and 'strong' postmodernism (Benhabib 1992: 213–25), 'a postmodernism of resistance' and 'a postmodernism of reaction' (Foster 1983: xi), progressive versus reactionary appropriations (Girroux 1990: 16) and affirmative and sceptical postmodernisms (Rosenau 1992: 15).

In this book, we side with those expressions of postmodern thinking that do not totally abandon the values of modernity and the Enlightenment project of human emancipation. Only 'strong' or 'extreme' forms of postmodern theory reject normative criticism and the usefulness of any forms of commonality underlying diversity. We believe that a 'weak' form of postmodernism informed by critical theory can contribute effectively to the construction of an emancipatory politics concerned with political action and social justice.

Thus what we call postmodern critical theory is concerned with political struggles against racism, sexism and colonialism. It is a postmodern approach that values diversity and legitimates difference. The chapters by Bob Pease, Lee FitzRoy and Karen Crinall address the problem of difference in specific ways. Bob explores the possibilities of a postmodern critical analysis in developing an understanding of men's (multiple) subjectivities, a body of thinking which has been little addressed by feminist theorising. Lee points to the need to recognise (and understand) experiences which do not superficially fit politically correct categories (women's violence against women), and suggests ways in which a postmodern feminist approach might begin to help us tackle the issue. Karen's chapter shows how traditional emancipatory approaches can inappropriately construct a victim identity for young women, and therefore how a postmodern feminism might help us work more effectively to resist the victimising process.

We acknowledge, along with Stainton and Swift (1996: 87), that if the concept of difference is to be useful in social work, it will need to recognise power and oppression. Leonard (1997) defines postmodern critical politics as a reconstructed project of emancipation. Rather than being at the end of emancipation, struggles against domination continue under changed historical conditions (1997: xiii). Karen Healy's chapter elucidates this issue of how power might be reconceptualised under these changed historical conditions. She targets the problem of how power is conceptualised in traditional modernist activist approaches, pointing to how power and identity have become frozen into oppositional categories, potentially reducing the possibilities for dialogue, interaction and change.

In this book, we would agree with Leonard's (1997) argument that the emancipatory project still continues, even though historical conditions change. The reconstructed emancipatory project, in particular, must involve changed epistemologies, as well as changes in material conditions, for this then will enable changes in both the internalised and externalised constructions of power relations.

DECONSTRUCTING TRADITIONAL SOCIAL WORK

Deconstruction is a method developed by Derrida (1976) for reading a text in such a way that the conceptual premises upon which the text is based are shown to fail by demonstrating how they are used inconsistently within the text itself. Sarap (1988: 60) argues that it is an attempt to dismantle the logic by which ideas and practices gain power and force. The suggestion is that all arguments contain certain key premises and that one can never escape this. Over time, the acceptance of the original premises becomes so powerful that one can barely think of the argument in any other way (Parker and Shotter 1990: 7).

Deconstruction is a series of techniques which enable one to identify and make visible the original hidden premises. Such techniques enable us to envisage ways of disrupting the dominant discourse and constructing positions of resistance (Parker and Shotter 1990: 209). In this way, deconstruction can be a method of radical political analysis. It can be used to critique ideologies that reproduce dominant relations of power (Ryan 1982: 38). Jan Fook's chapter develops the idea of deconstruction as critical reflexivity, and shows how such an approach can be used educationally (and in practice) to improve and change practice along emancipatory lines. It can thus be argued that the use of critical reflexivity helps achieve one of the purposes of postmodern critical social work, which is to deconstruct the truth claims of traditional social work (Brown 1994: 36). Peter Camilleri's chapter, in particular, deconstructs the traditional social work propensity to rely on scientistic claims regarding professional knowledge and expertise. He neatly analyses the oppositional categorising of 'theory and practice' in this way, and proposes new ways of building partnerships between providers and consumers of services, based on a postmodern critical approach.

CRITICAL SOCIAL WORK AS A COUNTER DISCOURSE

Another important element in constructing a postmodern critical practice is the concept of discourse. Foucault (1980: 93) defined discourses as 'historically variable ways of specifying knowledge and truth—what it is possible to speak at a given moment'. They specify sets of rules and the function of these rules is to define what is or is not the case. Thus the vocabulary of discourses allows choices to be made only within its own rules.

Discourse analysis examines the assumptions, language and myths that underpin particular positions in order to show that discursive practices are ordered according to underlying codes and rules which govern what may be thought or said at any time (Tilley 1990: 290). For example, socio-biology as a discourse shapes notions of what constitutes normal masculinity and femininity by arguing that certain meanings are the true ones (Weedon 1987: 130). Often, the prevailing view is only able to prevail because people are unaware that it is only one of several possible alternative views. Certainly, in this way, the dominant discourse of science has silenced the experiences of women and ethnic groups. Dominant discourses involve processes of domination whereby the oppressed often collude with the oppressor, taking for granted their discourse and their definition of the situation (Gitlin 1989:106).

In this context, social work is a discourse (Stevenson 1993). The social work discourse defines what a client is and what a social worker is. It also lays down rules for how they are to interact. The idea of 'social work' knowledge excludes other knowledge as being irrelevant and it constrains social workers to a particular knowledge base.

The important question for social work, then, is this: To what extent does social work remain a discourse based on the belief in the existence of objective professional knowledge (Leonard 1994: 24)? Alternatively, to what extent is it able to explore other accounts, histories and experiences? Linda Briskman and Carolyn Noble explore this question in relation to codes of ethics in social work, and try to pose some new models which are more inclusive of diversity. Lister Bainbridge looks at these questions in relation to the mental health field, and anlayses how particular perspectives have become dominant, and others marginalised, in our understanding of, and service provision in, the field of mental health.

Marxists and feminist materialists argue that discourses are not autonomous from social relations (Callinicos 1985: 87). They maintain that there are real institutional bases to these processes—for example, the economy and patriarchal social relations. Capitalist relations of production continue to be the central organising features of Western society. Commodity production and wage labour for capital still exist and workers are still dominated and exploited (Kellner 1989: 177). Also, women's oppression is not purely ideological or discursive; it also constitutes a specific material oppression (Moi 1985: 147). Thus, from a materialist perspective, discourses can be understood as part of the ideological apparatus which operates to legitimate the social order.

As critical theorists, we acknowledge that discourses represent political interests and that the most powerful discourses in our society have institutional bases in law (Weedon 1987: 41, 109). The recognition of discourse as a dimension of the real does not lead us to abandon attempts at understanding an extra-discursive reality (Woodiwiss 1990: 28).

However, the liberatory potential of Foucault's notion of discourse is that it provides the possibility of creating alternative discourses and repositioning ourselves in the dominant discourses. Personal and social change comes about by unravelling the discursive power of dominant discourses and re-creating ourselves as the basis for a collective politics of the future.

Discourses make positions available for individuals and these positions are taken up in relation to other people. When taken up, the world is seen from the standpoint of that position and this process involves, among other things, positioning oneself in relation to categories and story lines. It also involves locating oneself as a member of various sub-classes of categories as distinct from others. So one develops a sense of oneself 'as belonging to the world in certain ways and thus seeing the world from the perspective of one so positioned' (Davies and Harre 1990: 46–47). Through this process, people can become *fixed* in a position as they are shaped by 'the range of linguistic practices available to them to make sense' of the world (Potter and Wetherall 1987: 109).

The individual is thus constituted and reconstituted through a variety of discursive practices and changing material circumstances. This challenges the humanist conception of the subject as a freely choosing individual (John 1994: 59). Like Marshall (1994:

117), we find the concept of positionality useful in bringing 'together both subjectivity and structure as they converge in the individual'. Helen Jessup and Steve Rogerson illustrate how a combination of Foucauldian analysis and Freirian educational principles can be used in teaching an interpersonal communication practice which links both personal and structural change.

The relevance of this notion, which couples discursive constructions and material conditions for emancipatory social work practice, is that people can reconstitute themselves through a self-conscious and critically reflective practice. Individuals can reject the way in which they are positioned in discourse and can work towards the creation of new, more emancipatory, discourses, which have both internalised and externalised expressions.

To date, postmodern social work literature has focused more particularly on deconstructing the social work profession, its theory, practice and contexts. Now, though, it is the detailed connections between postmodern thinking and social work practice possibilities, particularly the more concrete and specific applications, that require further discussion. As well, further articulation is needed of the ways in which this fits with the emancipatory tradition of social work, established nearly three decades ago. How can social work be practised, from both a critical and a postmodern perspective? Each chapter in this volume addresses a specific aspect of this question.

TOWARDS POSTMODERN EMANCIPATORY PRACTICES IN SOCIAL WORK

The book has been organised along the following lines. Part I, 'Deconstructing the professional and organisational context of social work', begins the book with chapters which focus on the broader theoretical debates about social work and its context. Peter Camilleri conducts a comprehensive analysis of social work, including its own theoretical constructions, and the constructions of the context in which it operates. Gary Hough looks particularly at the organisational context in which social work is practised, deconstructs organisational and managerial imperatives, and points to the need to develop models for more responsive practice.

Part II, 'Dealing with diversity and difference', includes chapters which explore how the postmodern concepts of diversity and difference point to a reconceptualisation of practice in particular areas. Linda Briskman and Carolyn Noble criticise codes of ethics for their inability to acknowledge social and cultural differences, and try to formulate some directions which critical postmodern codes might take. Lee FitzRoy poses one of the major problematics in postmodern thinking for feminists: how to recognise and understand the experience of women in the area of assault which does not fit the norm. Karen Crinall looks at how our notions of difference need to recognise that the identity of 'victimhood' does not necessarily fit with the notions of selfhood which young women hold, and explores how this realisation can improve our practice with young women. Bob Pease ends this section by deconstructing the category of men, and demonstrating how a recognition of variations among men is central for understanding men's lives, and for reconstructing subjectivities and practices.

In Part III, 'Rethinking critical practice', Karen Healy begins by showing how activist social work practice has rested on a politics of identity which is potentially problematic for the emancipatory project, in that the possibilities for dialogue between 'powerful' and 'powerless' have been limited. Mary Lane develops the implications of aspects of postmodern thinking, such as diversity and uncertainty, and examines how they can be translated into transformative agendas in community development practice. Stephen Parker, Jan Fook and Bob Pease end this section by revisiting the concept of empowerment, which is central to emancipatory practice, and redeveloping it along postmodern critical lines.

In Part IV, 'Reconstructing social work education', Helen Jessup and Steve Rogerson begin by demonstrating how critical postmodern ideas can be enacted at the interpersonal communication level. Using Foucault's notion of discourse analysis and Freire's principles of liberatory education, they develop an approach to teaching interpersonal skills which allows the connection of personal and social change. Lister Bainbridge explores how the binary oppositional thinking inherent in modernist approaches to mental health can be challenged in the education process. Jan Fook ends this section by describing and developing the links between critical reflection and postmodern critical theory, and illustrates how the reflective process can be used as a method of teaching to improve practice.

The final section of the book, 'Critically interrogating the postmodern', concludes this study by raising questions, and engaging in debate about, the future of the postmodern critical approach in social work. The first chapter, by Jim Ife, raises doubts about the dangerously relativist tendencies of postmodern thinking. Ife argues for a reaffirmation of critical theory in rescuing the notions of social justice, human rights and structural oppression. In the final chapter, 'Emancipatory social work for a postmodern future', Jan Fook and Bob Pease respond to these criticisms, and summarise and discuss problematic themes and issues which arise from the chapters in the book.

Transforming Social Work Practice is intended as a contribution to the ongoing development of a practice and politics which is enabling, flexible and relevant. It does not attempt to resolve all the conflicts and debates about postmodern critical social work, but rather aims to air them, and to provide examples of thinking which might transform our practice through a recognition and incorporation of the dilemmas into our experience. We hope this is the spirit in which you will read the book and receive the ideas within it.

NOTE

1. Although we use the term 'postmodern critical social work' to describe the framework we are advancing, we have not been prescriptive about this with our contributors. Thus some of our contributors use a variety of different designations to describe the intersection of critical theory, postmodernism and progressive social work.

REFERENCES

Argyris, C. and Schon, D. (1976) *Theory in Practice: Increasing Professional Effectiveness*, Addison-Wesley, Massachusetts

Bailey, R. and Brake, M. (eds) (1980) *Radical Social Work and Practice*, Edward Arnold, London

——(eds) (1975) *Radical Social Work*, Edward Arnold, London

Benhabib, S. (1992) *Situating the Self: Gender, Community and Postmodernism*, Polity Press, Cambridge

Brook, E. and Davis, A. (eds) (1985) *Women, the Family and Social Work*, Tavistock, London

Brown, C. (1994) 'Feminist Postmodernism and the Challenge of Diversity', in A. Chambon and A. Irving (eds), *Essays on Postmodernism and Social Work*, Canadian Scholars' Press, Toronto.

Burman, E., Aitkin, G., Alldred, P., Allwood, R., Billington, T., Goldberg, B., Gordon Lopez, A., Heenan, C., Marks, D., Warner, S. (eds) (1996) *Psychology Discourse Practice*, Taylor and Francis, London

Callinicos, A. (1985) 'Postmodernism, Poststructuralism, Post Marxism?', *Theory, Culture and Society*, vol. 2, no. 3, pp. 85–101

Camilleri, P. (1996) *Reconstructing Social Work*, Abebury, Aldershot

Cohen, S. (1975) 'It's Alright for you to Talk', in R. Bailey and M. Brake (eds), *Radical Social Work*, Edward Arnold, London, pp. 76–95

Corrigan, P. and Leonard, P. (1978) *Social Work Practice Under Capitalism: A Marxist Approach*, Macmillan, London

Davies, B. and Harre, R. (1990) 'Positioning: The Discursive Production of Selves', *Journal for the Theory of Social Behaviour*, vol. 20, no. 1, pp. 43–63

De Maria, W. (1993) 'Exploring Radical Social Work Teaching in Australia', *Journal of Progressive Human Services*, vol. 4, no. 2, pp. 45–63

Derrida, J. (1976) *Of Grammatology*, John Hopkins University Press, London

Dominelli, L. and Mcleod, E. (1989) *Feminist Social Work*, Macmillan, London

Featherstone, B. and Fawcett, B. (1995) 'Oh No! Not More "isms"', *Social Work Education*, vol. 14, no. 3, pp. 25–43

Fook, J. (1993) *Radical Casework: A Theory of Practice*, Allen & Unwin, Sydney

——(ed.) (1996) *The Reflective Researcher: Social Workers' Theories of Practice Research*, Allen & Unwin, Sydney

Foster, H. (1983) 'Postmodernism: A Preface', in H. Foster (ed.), *Postmodern Culture*, Pluto Press, London

Foucault, M. (1980) *Power/Knowledge: Selected Interviews and Other Writings 1972–1977*, Pantheon Books, New York

Galper, J. (1975) *The Politics of Social Services*, Prentice Hall, Englewood Cliffs

——(1980) *Social Work Practice: A Radical Perspective*, Prentice-Hall, Englewood Cliffs

Girroux, H. (1990) *Curriculum Discourse as Postmodernist Practice*, Deakin University Press, Geelong

Gitlin, T. (1989) 'Postmodernism: Roots and Politics', *Dissent*, Winter, pp. 100–108

Grinnell, R. (1988) *Social Work Research and Evaluation*, F.E. Peacock, Itasca

Harre Hindmarsh, J. (1992) *Social Work Oppositions*, Avebury, Aldershot

Hartman, A. (1990) 'Many Ways of Knowing', *Social Work*, vol. 35, no. 1, pp. 3–4

——(1991) 'Words Create Worlds', *Social Work*, vol. 36, no. 4, pp. 275–76

——(1992) 'In Search of Subjugated Knowledge', *Social Work*, vol. 37, no. 6, 483–84

Haworth, G. (1991) 'My Paradigm Can Beat Your Paradigm: Some Reflections on Knowledge Conflicts', *Journal of Sociology and Social Welfare*, vol. XVIII, Dec., pp. 35–50

Healy, B. and Fook, J. (1994) 'Reinventing Social Work', in J. Ife, S. Leitman and P. Murphy (eds), *Advances in Social Work and Welfare Education*, AASWWE, University of Western Australia, pp. 42–55

Healy, K. (1995) 'Rethinking Power in Activist Social Work', unpublished paper presented at the National Australian Association of Social Workers Conference, Launceston, July

Ife, J. (1996) *Rethinking Social Work: Towards Critical Practice*, Longman, Melbourne

Irving, A. (1994) 'Feminist Postmodernism and the Challenge of Diversity', in A. Chambon and A. Irving (eds), *Essays on Postmodernism and Social Work*, Canadian Scholars' Press, Toronto

Irwin, J., Larbelestier, J. and Wilkinson, M. (1994) 'Social Work Education, Resistance and Change', in K.E.H. Hesser (ed.), *Social Work Education: State of the Art*, Official Congress Publication, 27th Congress of the International Association of Schools of Social Work, Amsterdam, pp. 147–52

John, L. (1994) 'Borrowed Knowledge in Social Work: An Introduction to Post-Structuralism and Postmodernity', in A. Chambon and A. Irving (eds) *Essays on Postmodernism and Social Work*, Canadian Scholars' Press, Toronto

Kellner, D. (1989) *Critical Theory, Marxism and Modernity*, Basil Blackwell, Oxford

Laird, J. (ed.) (1993) *Revisioning Social Work Education*, Haworth, New York

Langan, M. and Lee, P. (eds) (1989) *Radical Social Work Today*, Unwin Hyman, London

Leonard, P. (1994) 'Knowledge/Power and Postmodernism: Implications for the Practice of a Critical Social Work Education', *Canadian Social Work Review*, vol. 11, no. 1, pp. 11–26

——(1997) *Postmodern Welfare: Reconstructing an Emancipatory Project*, Sage, London

Marchant, H. and Wearing, B. (eds) (1986) *Gender Reclaimed*, Hale & Iremonger, Sydney

Marshall, B. (1994) *Engendering Modernity*, Polity Press, Cambridge

Moi, T. (1985) *Sexual/Textual Politics*, Routledge, New York

Moreau, M. (1979) 'A structural approach to social work practice', *Canadian Journal of Social Work Education*, vol. 5, no. 1, pp. 78–94

——(1990) 'Empowerment Through Advocacy and Consciousness-Raising: Implication of a Structural Approach to Social Work, *Journal of Sociology and Social Welfare*, vol. 17, no. 2, pp. 53–67

Mullaly, B. (1993) *Structural Social Work: Ideology, Theory and Practice*, McClelland and Stewart, Toronto

——(1998) *Structural Social Work: Ideology, Theory and Practice*, Oxford University Press, Toronto

Pardeck, J.T., Murphy, J.W. and Choi, J.M. (1994) 'Some Implications of Postmodernism for Social Work Practice', *Social Work*, vol. 39, no. 4, pp. 343–46

Parker, I. and Shotter, J. (1990) 'Introduction', *Deconstructing Social Psychology*, (ed.) I. Parker and J. Shotter, Routledge, London

Parry, A. and Doan, R. (1994) *Story Revisions: Narrative Therapy in the Postmodern World*, The Guilford Press, New York

Parton, N. (1994) 'Problematics of Government, (Post)modernity, and Social Work, *British Journal of Social Work*, vol. 24, pp. 9–32

——(1996) (ed.) *Social Theory, Social Change and Social Work*, Routledge, London

Payne, M. (1997) *Modern Social Work Theory*, Macmillan, London

Pease, B. (1987) Towards a Socialist Praxis in Social Work. Unpublished Master of Behavavioural Science thesis, La Trobe University, Melbourne, 1987

——(1990) 'Towards Collaborative Research on Socialist Theory and Practice in Social Work', *Social Change and Social Welfare Practice*, R. Thorpe and J. Petruchenia (eds), Hale and Iremonger, Sydney

——(1996) Reforming Men: Masculine Subjectivities and the Politics and Practices of Profeminism. Unpublished PhD thesis, La Trobe University, Melbourne

Piele, C. and McCouat, M. (1997) 'The Rise of Relativism: The Future of Theory and Knowledge Development in Social Work', *British Journal of Social Work*, vol. 27, pp. 343–60

Potter, J. and Wetherall, M. (1987) *Discourse and Social Psychology,* Sage, London

Pozatek, E. (1994) 'The Problem of Certainty: Clinical Social Work in the Postmodern Era', *Social Work*, vol. 39, no. 4, pp. 396–403

Ristock, J. and Pennell, J. (1996) *Community Research as Empowerment: Feminist Links, Postmodern Interruptions,* Oxford University Press, Toronto

Rojek, C., Peacock, G. and Collins, S. (1988) *Social Work and Received Ideas,* Routledge, London

Rosenau, P. (1992) *Postmodernism and the Social Sciences,* Princeton University Press, Princeton

Rossiter, A. (1996) 'A Perspective on Critical Social Work', *Journal of Progressive Human Services,* vol. 7, no. 2, pp. 23–41

Ryan, M. (1982) *Marxism and Deconstruction: A Critical Articulation*, John Hopkins University Press, Baltimore

Sarup, M. (1992) *An Introductory Guide to Poststructuralism and Postmodernism*, Harvester Wheatsheaf, London

Smith, C. and White, S. (1997) 'Parton, Howe and Postmodernity: A Critical Comment on Mistaken Identity', *British Journal of Social Work*, vol. 27, pp. 275–95

Solas, J. (1996) *The (De)Construction of Educational Practice in Social Work*, Avebury, Aldershot

Stainton, T. and Swift, K. (1996) ' "Difference" and Social Work Curriculum', *Canadian Social Work Review,* vol. 13, no. 1, pp. 75–90

Stevenson, K. (1993) 'Social Work Discourse and the Social Work Interview', *Economy and Society,* vol. 22, no. 1, pp. 42–75

Taylor-Gooby, P. (1994) 'Postmodernism and Social Policy: A Great Leap Backwoods', *Journal of Social Policy*, vol. 23, no. 3, pp. 385–404

Thompson, N. (1993) *Anti-Discriminatory Practice*, Macmillan, London

Throssell, H. (1975) (ed.) *Social Work: Radical Essays*, University of Queensland Press, St Lucia

Tilley, C. (1990) 'M. Foucault: Towards an Archealogy of Archealogy', in C. Tilley (ed.), *Reading Material Culture: Structuralism, Hermeneutics, Post Structuralism*, Basil Blackwell, Oxford

Weedon, C. (1987) *Feminist Practice and Post Structuralist Theory,* Basil Blackwell, Oxford

White, M. (1995) *Re-Authoring Lives: Interviews and Essays,* Dulwich Centre, Adelaide

White, M. and Epston, D. (1989) *Literate Means to Therapeutic Ends,* Dulwich Centre, Adelaide

Woodiwiss, A. (1990) *Social Theory After Feminism,* Pluto Press, London

PART I

Deconstructing the professional and organisational context of social work

2 Social work and its search for meaning: Theories, narratives and practices
Peter Camilleri

INTRODUCTION: IS THERE A BEGINNING?

This chapter grew out of a personal crisis. After ten years as a practitioner, I was struck with a sense of uncertainty about social work. After drifting into academia essentially as a sociologist and then as a social work lecturer, I spent the next decade teaching, arguing and writing about the social work discourse. Embarking on a doctoral program gave me the opportunity to be self-indulgent and focus on what it is that constitutes social work. As a sociologist, as well as a social worker, I took it as axiomatic that all action is theory driven. I accepted the ethnomethodological position that we are all 'sociologists'—that is, not only do we question the world around us, but we also theorise about why things happen and how they happen. Theory had a comfortable feel to it in terms of the sociological literature. However, once I turned to social work, theory seemed to take on a different meaning and social work was continually exhorting itself to use theory in practice. From a sociological position, practice was theoretical action and, in Weberian terms, action was meaningful behaviour. Problematically theory was used in the singular and, as Beilharz (1991: 1) notes:

> Theory is useful; it enables, it helps us better to understand what we already knew, intuitively, in the first place. But theory is always plural, *theories*, and multicentred.

During this period of self-indulgence, social work itself was going through a crisis and the number of texts outlining this crisis, such as Brewer and Lait (1980) and Clarke et al. (1980) were indicating a crisis in confidence affecting not only the sponsors of social work but also social workers themselves. This crisis was an echo of the general malaise facing the social sciences and the welfare state. The social sciences during the 1970s and 1980s had embarked on a period of a highly developed systematic and synethic theorising (Beilharz 1991). These were attempts to develop comprehensive theories to account for exploitation and domination. The new social movements such as feminism, indigenous rights, environmentalism, rights of the disabled were challenging the discourse of the social sciences. These 'voices' were demanding that they be heard.

For social work, the crisis was both internal and external. The external crisis was in the relationship between social work and the welfare state. The transformation of the welfare state has seen social work become more marginalised as the ideological framework for services and programs has shifted significantly to contracting out services through competitive tendering. Social work has been challenged by this new managerialism and finds itself uncomfortably located in the welfare state. Social work's future is uncertain and the values it holds appear to be under constant attack and threat.

During the 1970s and 1980s, social work also experienced a considerable degree of crisis, in particular in terms of uncertainty of what constitutes practice in social work. The tension emerged between social work as a scientific activity and as art or humanist endeavour. This tension can creatively be seen as social work practice being in the process of transformation between its modernist origins and its struggle in a postmodernist arena.

MODERNISM AND POSTMODERNISM: FRAMING THE PROBLEMATIC

The argument put forward by sociologists such as Harvey (1989) and Crook et al. (1992) is that we are experiencing a societal transformation from modernity to a radically different form of society tentatively described as postmodern. Transformation is occurring at the economic, social and cultural levels (Crook et al. 1992: 1–40). For social work, the experience of this transformation has been evident in the changing nature of the welfare state and the concerns about what constitutes the practice of social work.

For many social workers, the adjective 'postmodern', which is now increasingly used in social work texts, appears to throw them into the middle of a conversation. There is a sense of everyone knowing what is going on except them. It is a conversation constructed in a language that is at best obtuse and at worst incomprehensible. It appears designed to produce confusion. It is perhaps inevitable that a 'space' needs to be created to take the reader from the certainties embedded in modernity to a new discourse in which uncertainty, fragmentation and local and contingent knowledge are central.

Social work can be located within modernity. This means that social work is characterised by an emphasis on rationality and scientific knowledge. It has involved the development of a worldview in which logic and science are brought to bear on explaining and controlling problematic people and situations. Modernism involves dichotomies—for example, reason is elevated above emotion (Gorman 1993: 248). Postmodernism involves a shift and moving beyond the notion of dichotomies; it challenges the very notions of certainty, objectivity and worldviews, stripping away the notion of grand narratives which attempt to develop general, abstract and timeless axioms (Fook 1995).

Scientific discourse has been about things and facts, and hence has seen itself as located outside the phenomenon so that it can comment authoritatively (Game 1991). However, such discourses discursively construct the phenomenon they purport to objectively study. The implications for social science have been to locate the researcher within the research, to question the notion of rigid disciplinary boundaries, to shift emphasis and explore the unique, the local and the everyday (Smith 1987).

For me, the problematic is to develop a critical framework in which social work can respond to the challenges of postmodernism. I agree with Fook's (1995) view that social work is about social justice. However, social justice is not a universal, timeless and absolute concept. We need to pose the following question continually: How do we further social justice principles in this particular situation? (Fook 1995: 10).

SOCIAL WORK THEORY: SENSE AND MEANING

The history of social work theory is essentially a story of a search for coherence. Social work has been seeking a grand theory—or, in postmodern terms, a metanarrative. This metanarrative is an attempt to provide practitioners, consumers and sponsors alike with a sense of coherence about what constitutes the practices of social work, how social work engages in its practices and who benefits from such practices. Social work has been unrelenting in its search for such a metanarrative.

The theories of social work are not just treated as givens and resources, but they constitute the discourse of social work.

Theories are not just there as contextual resources, but are in part an aspect of social work itself. The texts of social work provide histories of social work, theories and models of practice, arguments on the nature of research and practice in social work and a connection between and across national boundaries and times. They are a powerful discourse in which individuals can locate themselves and their practices. We need to see these texts not just as a resource for the context on social work, but as a topic for analysis.

Social work texts treat the written word as theory. The word is seen and treated as 'theory', so to be theory means to be written. What this does for the discourse of social work is to treat all written texts as the 'theory' of social work. A number of writers such as Howe (1987), Payne (1997) and Roberts (1990) have noted the difficulty that this provides for understanding social work as a social practice. Roberts (1990: 15–48), in particular, explores the notion of 'theory' as used in the social work discourse. He notes the conflagration of terms such as 'theory', 'concepts', 'frameworks', 'models', 'approaches' and 'paradigms' in the social work literature. Social work texts often use these terms interchangeably. For practitioners, the problematic nature of theory in which theory is bracketed with a range of intellectual activities derides their 'doing' of social work. 'Doing' is separated from 'knowing'. The divide between 'theory' and 'practice' is an important theoretical problem.

The search for and development of a unifying theory of social work has been accomplished in the context of a series of crises. The notion of a 'generic' integrated approach to social work practice has been as a response to a number of crises. The history of theory development in social work has been forged in the challenges of practice, the location of the practitioner in organisations and the emergence of a radical critique. The overriding purpose of theory in social work has been to demonstrate the coherence and unity of the practice. Theory, it is argued, has been about creating an 'ideal' rather than providing practitioners with an understanding of their actions.

In this chapter, I expand upon social work's search for a unifying theory. In the following section, the argument concerning the problematic of theory and practice is outlined. I argue that the theory and practice dichotomy is of little relevance. Social work is about 'doing' and it is that doing/acting/knowledge that constitutes social work. I then move the argument on to examining the metaphor of the two 'voices' of social work. This highlights the divergent paths social work can be constructed around. These 'voices' provide for a very different vision of social work practice.

They are conceptualised as 'social work as science' and social work as 'art or humanistic endeavour'. The chapter then concludes with an alternative vision of social work, which allows for the empowering of the individual, community and practitioner. The transformation of the welfare state provides a small opening for the development of radical and empowering strategies for individuals and communities.

THE PROBLEMATIC OF 'UNIFYING' SOCIAL WORK

Social work's search for a 'unifying' theory to explain and provide for its practice has been the feature of what can be termed 'academic' social work (Meyer 1983). This discourse is evident in the texts and provides for a re-reading in which the apparent tensions and contradictions between what is termed 'theory' and 'practice' can be 'unpacked'. For many commentators, the so-called 'divide' between theory and practice is not about the problematic of translating *a* theory into *a* practice, but about the politics of the occupation (Pilalis 1986). In essence, who is to control the discourse of social work: the academics or the practitioners? It is this tension, this dialectic, that produces, transmits and reproduces the discourse of social work.

The literature discusses theory and practice as separate activities and hence as problematical. A number of writers, such as Pithouse (1987) and Sibeon (1991), have noted the strong 'oral' culture of social work practitioners; others, such as Sheldon (1978), talk about the development of two distinct subcultures in social work: the 'theoretical subculture' and the much larger 'practice subculture'. A 'theoretical subculture' is located in universities and colleges and a much larger 'practice subculture' exists amongst practitioners. Sheldon argues that this latter culture does not use or recognise the importance of research. The practitioners have seen the work of academics as having little relevance to their world of practice. In the social work literature, the profession and the academics continually debate the question of practice versus theory. It is argued by some that the theory and practice of social work are separate activities which, in the final analysis, have very little to do with each other (Goldstein 1986).

The theory and practice problematic of social work is based on the premise that theory and practice have similar purposes. However, it can be argued that theory itself—or at least its development and propagation—occurs within academic institutions and is consequently a social practice. In examining social work 'theory', the literature appears to use it in a rather ambiguous way.

The theory–practice divide has been 'read' at a number of different levels. For example, in Payne's (1997) comprehensive text, he argues that there are essentially four levels of theories in social work: theories about social work; theories of social work; theories that are contextual for social work; and theories of social work's practice and method. The simplistic debate of the original theory–practice argument has led to a greater appreciation of the complexity of what constitutes both theory and practice within social work. Smid and Van Krieken (1984) make the salient point that we need to think in terms of theories and practices. The emphasis on a theory and a practice has demonstrated the essential unity of social work. However, that has been problematic for social work: it has become more apparent that the search for and development of 'theory' has decontextualised the practices in which social workers engage. To connect practice to context would be to acknowledge the fragmentation of social work and the possibility of social work being constituted in different forms.

Social work theory has seen a massive explosion of models and frameworks since the 1960s. According to Germain (1983), before the 1960s there were only three major approaches to social casework, with the third approach only appearing in 1957 as an attempt to unite the other competing theories. By 1983, Germain could identify fifteen separate and distinct 'practice approaches'.

> With one exception, all formulations examined, as well as others
> not examined, have been proposed and developed by
> university-based social work educators . . . It leads us to ask how
> much university-based social workers talk only to one another in
> formulating practice approaches. Do their formulations reflect the
> activities of Practice? (1983: 55)

These American theoretical developments may be an outcome of academic practices. The demands of tenure put social work academics into a situation of needing to constantly publish (Karger 1983). For social work in particular, there is a need to demonstrate to its constant critics its scientific status and hence to be able to claim academic validity (Karger 1983; Sibeon 1991). These developments have been occurring at a time of crisis within the welfare state and it could be argued that they are symptomatic of the fragmentation of that welfare state.

Academic social workers are important for the profession since they attempt to provide its credibility. This is done through the production of theories. It would appear as though the two activities—theory production and the 'oral' culture of social work practice—are in tension. However, the social work discourse is constructed from a large 'oral' culture, which is discursively produced as a reading of the texts of social work. Its meaning and coherence depends on the texts of social work.

A metatheory was needed to incorporate all the possibilities of social work into a coherent whole. Researchers in social work were wanting to demonstrate the 'scientific' basis of practice (see Bloom and Fischer 1982; Ivanoff et al. 1987; Karger 1983; Peile 1988). In the American social work journals of the 1980s, there was an ongoing, major and interesting debate. It concerned the claims of social work to be either a scientific practice or a humanist endeavour. The next section explores the debate and the issues it raised about the nature of social work.

THE 'VOICES' OF SOCIAL WORK: IS IT A 'SCIENCE' OR IS IT 'ART'?

Mirroring the theory–practice divide, and in some sense constituted by that debate has been often a series of bitter and fiercely contested claims in the literature of social work as either a science or a humanist endeavour. The concern of the academic-researcher was that, as the social work enterprise became institutionalised within academia, the rules and conventions governing that social world would necessitate social work becoming more 'scientific'. For academic-researchers, this meant that practitioners would utilise research findings; that the academic social workers would provide the 'questions' for the profession; and that theory development was the cornerstone of the discipline.

The theme of social work research is empiricism. The message of the discourse, however, has contested that social work is about 'real' and objective social problems that are constituted within and through discursively produced 'subjects'. The methodological implication of the normative consensus perspective was empiricism. The debate concerning the scientific status of research which took place in American journals such as the *Social Service Review* and *Social Casework* during the late 1970s and throughout the 1980s demonstrates the powerful tradition of empiricism in social work. Empiricism constructs a 'real' world in which 'things' can be measured and known. Difficulties that arise are due to either lack of sophisticated measuring techniques or operational inadequacies (Heineman 1981). The empirical validation of social work addresses two major issues: first, a model of professionalism; and second, the issue of accountability. The emphasis on positivist research methods has been a response to the professionalising project of social work, with the search for 'scientific respectability' an ongoing concern.

The literature has sparked opposition among a number of writers, who have predicated their response to the empiricism of social researchers-academics on humanism (see Carew 1987; England 1986; Goldstein 1990). Social work within this tradition rejects empiricism and sees social work as 'art'. The push for an alternative research paradigm has been well noted in the literature over the last fifteen years. American academics such as Goldstein (1990), Heineman (1981), Imre (1984), Marsh (1983), Piper (1989) and Weick (1987) have constantly called for a non-positivist research paradigm in which the practice of social work is the core of research and provides for the 'questions' to be asked.

In the literature, there have been often bitter and angry responses by researchers in the empirical tradition to this call for an alternative paradigm. Though the call for the use of qualitative methods and naturalistic inquiry has been widespread, little discernible change in the social work discourse has occurred. Empiricism *is* the tradition of social work research and the questions raised by postmodernism have had little impact.

Davis (1985) argues that the conflict is about competing worlds. A reading of these two worldviews is that they represent two distinctive 'voices'. The mainly 'masculine' culture of the academic world relies on a world that is 'rational, reasonable and abstract'. The world of practice is mainly a 'feminine' one in which 'knowing, caring and doing' are bounded up with each other in a complex interaction.

> Those who have created and affirmed the meanings in academic social work have been primarily a community of men, whereas those who have created and affirmed meanings in the world of practice have been primarily women . . . Whereas women's mode of thinking is contextual and narrative, men's is abstract and formal . . . The voice of women has not been limited to concern with caring in a relationship. It has also been expressed in contextual and narrative approaches to social work practice . . . The female voice in social work has also been expressed through reliance on and valuing of intuition. (Davis 1985 107–9)

The recognition of the 'female' voice in social work is to fold back the world of academic social work within the practice of social work. The development of a critical perspective into which we challenge both ourselves and our clients into redesigning and transforming social relations is central to social work (see Ife 1997).

SOCIAL WORK AND WELFARE

Social work as a discourse is located within the sector of the economy and polity to do with welfare. The debate that social work has been submerged within over the last two decades has revolved around how and in what ways the welfare state is changing (Bryson 1992; Carney and Hanks 1994; Mishra 1984). Social work has become a distinct feature of the welfare state and welfare and social work are often synonymous terms. The practice of social work has also been transformed: where social workers practise and the sort of work they do are both extremely varied. For many critics, social work is straining to hold those activities together in one discourse (Wenocur and Reisch 1989).

Issues of privatisation, the rise of consumerism, the concern over professional power and its discourse, and the relationship between the state and its citizenry have shaped the debate over the welfare state. There are genuine implications for practitioners in this debate. Where they are to practise and in what ways they are to practise are being constructed in an active discourse between consumers, the state and community organisations (Yeatman 1994). The shape of the relationship between client and practitioner is being contested.

For practitioners, this transformation of welfare provides a sense of uncertainty of both social work and their personal place within that framework. The values that underpinned social work in the past, and that were characterised as part of the modernity project, are becoming more contested. Contingent and local decision-making are replacing the moral certainty of practice. Social workers feel adrift, and their expectations of what constitutes social work have been changed by their experiences in the welfare state.

Consumers of services and the funders of services want different things. While that is problematic for practitioners, as it is unclear what is required and contradictory demands are often placed on them, it is nevertheless something social workers have to deal with. The forging of a new relationship that incorporates different aspects and is constructed within a genuine respect for giving power and knowledge to recipients of service is still within the crucible of change. A new form of practice which is local and contextual, and linked to the politics of transformation, needs to be developed. This involves a very different sense of citizenship. The emerging relationship between the state and the citizens may well provide for a radical framework of practice.

SOCIAL WORK PRACTICE AND CITIZENSHIP

The crisis of consensus that characterised the last two decades in relationship to the welfare state has led to a renewal of ideas and social thought over the nature of citizenship. The dramatic and stringent discourse of the 'New Right', in which the welfare state—and by implication and at times explicitly—social work, was constructed as damaging the fabric of the individual, community and the economy, led to some vigorous defence of the welfare state (see Bean et al. 1985; Wilding 1986). In defending the welfare state, theorists were concerned not to fall into the trap of defending aspects of it that were damaging. There was a recognition that the welfare state was in need of significant overhaul—that the world had literally changed. The dynamics of a world economic order, the post-industrial nature of the international economy and the challenges to the motifs of authority have questioned the very possibility of a welfare state (Yeatman 1994).

Social welfare theorists have resurrected the notion of citizenship as the source of renewal for the welfare state. It is about developing a new 'social contract' between the citizenry and the state in the development and delivery of services. The state as the site of service delivery is fast disappearing. Its role as funder, contractor, regulator and evaluator continues to grow. The privatisation and corporatisation of services provides for a very different and potentially radical approach to services. For the recipients of such services, what is problematic is who is to control these. Recipients are subjected to these services rather than having their voices heard within the discourse. The acknowledgment of the rights of recipients with the introduction of *charters* of services, while providing for a framework of access and equity, does not deal with the problematic of need. Which voices are listened to when the emphasis on fiscal frugalness and competitiveness is engulfing the state is clearly problematic. The opening of what are somewhat loosely termed market forces to the delivery of human services has the potential to further construct recipients as 'objects' of services. There is a need for some agency to listen to the voices of the recipients and to clamour with those voices to be heard.

Professionals are necessary. Consumers of services recognise the value and expertise of the professional. Alternative strategies, in which both the skills and expertise of professionals and the paramount needs of consumers as the focus of service delivery are recognised, need to be implemented within a new partnership model. Writers such as Rees (1991), Rojek et al. (1988), and Weeks (1988) provide the beginnings of a discourse of practice in which practitioners and consumers are involved in a democratic relationship. The voices of both practitioners and consumers have to be heard.

> Professionals have to be trained to be accountable in these ways and consumers need to know that there are information and advocacy services they can call on if they need them. This partnership model actually privileges all the parties. It does not invert the usual relationship of professional domination by making the consumer, rather than the professional, top dog. Indeed, we should be wary of contemporary government policy which is making the consumer sovereign. By a relative marginalisation of professional knowledge (and a relative deprofessionalization of human services), governments are achieving a cheapening of services but are depriving consumers and carers of the contribution of expert knowledge to the process of defining and meeting their needs. (Yeatman 1994: 52)

The focus on citizenship within current social science discourse provides for new forms of practice of social work. Building on the work of Marshall (1950), social theorists and feminists have argued for a new and dynamic relationship between the state and its citizens (Turner 1993; Yeatman 1994). The state, as has been demonstrated by feminists, can be a site in which struggle and contest for rights can be intertwined with services (Yeatman 1994). The welfare state for practitioners has only recently been a site of practice. Social work was previously located within the residual and charity-sponsored section of service delivery. Social work is in a process of transformation. It needs to develop new models and methods of practice. This can be done without accepting the new managerialism. It is about putting people first and developing a genuine partnership.

The transformation of the welfare state provides the opportunity for social work to construct a new discourse. Both the politics of representation and politics of diversity that feminist theorists have argued for allow the other, the marginalised, to have their 'voices' heard and their needs acted upon (Yeatman 1994). The contested nature of the welfare state, in which services are either constructed as rights of citizens or as largesse of the state, is finely balanced.

The Left and the New Right have attacked the welfare state for its lack of choice and control of services. The solutions offered, however, are radically different. The New Right has seen the market as the most appropriate model for the satisfaction of human needs. Services are either being privatised or constructed within the model of the market and the service is mirrored on the private market 'fee for service' concept. As Yeatman (1994) has noted, the notion of consumer sovereignty is problematic. The marketplace does not provide for the Weberian notion of 'ethic of responsibility' (see Yeatman 1994: 98–99). The 'other'—those who are marginalised and the disadvantaged—will be swamped within the marketplace as they are now. Their voices will not be heard.

The possibilities of choice and control over the services they receive are, however, an aspect of market relations that are of value to a new partnership. The development of alternative services, which are embedded in a culture of individual choice and control, provides an opportunity for social work. Market relations can be eschewed within a discourse of exchange of services and goods. It is income generating rather than profit making. Holistic Health Centres and Feminist Therapy Centres offer services which are private and contractual. They are, however, modelled on choice and control. While these in themselves are marginal services and affect relatively few consumers, they are of interest in developing new strategies for social work. Choice and control are the key concepts within the new partnership. For social work practitioners, this will involve a new discourse; it will involve the development of what Yeatman (1994) calls 'emergent' strategies. The services that are developed will need to be local and continually changing to meet the expressed needs of radically divergent communities.

CONCLUSION

Social work as a practice is facing a transformation of the welfare state and its position is problematic. Social work is in *crisis*; its push for professional status has been at the expense of playing a determining role within the debate on the nature of the welfare state. It is in danger of becoming irrelevant.

Already in the last decade, we have seen the rise of new occupations within the Social and Community Services Sector, such as rehabilitation counsellors, community services workers and case managers. All these new developments are challenging social work's position within the welfare state. What is of most concern is not that they are unable to provide a quality service, but that practice is constructed within a discourse of rational and technical achievement. Social work, whatever its accomplishments, is constructed as a moral and political enterprise. Its value base paradoxically provides for uncertainty and possibilities of partnership with recipients of services (see Ife 1997). Social work does have a tradition in social justice; it is time to move from the rhetorical to the problematic of practice. This is about developing a language of practice which provides for a recognition of the skilful activity of the work and the 'empowering' of both the recipient and practitioner (Rees 1991). It is about developing new forms of organisation and practices.

Social work is a social practice. It is diverse and value-laden. These things are the basis on which new partnerships can be built. Risk and uncertainty will be the characteristic of social work practice in the coming decade.

REFERENCES

Bean, P., Ferris, J. and Whynes, D. (eds) (1985) *In Defence of Welfare*, Tavistock Publications, London

Beilharz, P. (ed.) (1991) *Social Theory*, Allen & Unwin, Sydney

Bloom, M. and Fisher, J. (1982) *Evaluating Practices: Guidelines for the Accountable Profession*, Prentice Hall, Englewood Cliffs, N.J.

Brewer, C. and Lait, J. (1980) *Can Social Work Survive?* Temple Smith, London

Bryson, L. (1992) *Welfare and the State*, Macmillan, London

Carew, R. (1987) 'The Place of Intuition in Social Work Activity', *Australian Social Work*, vol. 40, no. 3, pp. 5–10

Carney, T. and Hanks, P. (1994) *Social Security in Australia*, Oxford University Press, Melbourne

Clarke, J., Langan, M. and Lee, M. (1980) 'The Conditions of Crisis in Criminology', P. Carlen and M. Collison (eds), *Radical Issues in Criminology*, Martin Robertson, Oxford

Crook, S., Pakulski, J. and Waters, M. (1992) *Postmodernization: Change in Advanced Society*, Sage, London

Davis, L. (1985) 'Female and Male Voices in Social Work', *Social Work*, vol. 30, pp. 106–13

England, H. (1986) *Social Work as Art*, Allen & Unwin, London

Fook, J. (1995) 'Social Work: Asking the Relevant Questions', paper presented at the 24th National AASW Conference, Launceston

Game, A. (1991) *Undoing the Social: Towards a Deconstructive Sociology*, Open University Press, Milton Keynes

Germain, C. (1983) 'Technological Advances' in *Handbook of Clinical Social Work*, Jossey-Bass, San Franscisco

Goldstein, H. (1986) 'Toward the Integration of Theory and Practice: A Humanistic Approach', *Social Work*, vol. 31, pp. 352–57

——(1990) 'The Knowledge Base of Social Work Practice: Theory, Wisdom, Analogue, or Art?' *Families in Society*, vol. 71, pp. 32–43

Gorman, J. (1993) 'Postmodernism and the Conduct of Inquiry in Social Work', *Affilia*, vol. 8, no. 3, pp. 247–64

Harvey, D. (1989) *The Condition of Postmodernity*, Basil Blackwell, Oxford

Heineman, M. (1981) 'The Obsolete Scientific Imperative in Social Work Research', *Social Service Review*, vol. 55, pp. 371–97

Howe, D. (1987) *An Introduction to Social Work*, Wildwood House, Aldershot

Ife, J. (1997) *Rethinking Social Work: Towards Critical Practice*, Longman, Melbourne

Imre, R. (1984) 'The Nature of Knowledge in Social Work', *Social Work*, vol. 29, pp. 41–45

Ivanoff, A., Blythe, B. and Briar, S. (1987) 'The Empirical Clinical Practice Debate', *Social Casework*, vol. 68, May, pp. 290–98

Karger, H. (1983) 'Science, Research, and Social Work: Who Controls the Profession?', *Social Work*, vol. 28, pp. 200–205

Marsh, J. (1983) 'Research and Innovation in Social Work Practice: Avoiding the Headless Machine', *Social Service Review*, vol. 57, no. 4, pp. 582–98

Marshall, T. H. (1950) *Citizenship and Social Class and Other Essays*, Cambridge University Press, Cambridge

Meyer, C. (1983) 'The Search for Coherence', in *Clinical Social Work in the Eco-Systems Perspective*, Columbia University Press, New York

Mishra, R. (1984) *The Welfare State in Crisis*, Wheatsheaf Books, Brighton

Payne, M. (1997) *Modern Social Work Theory*, 2nd edn, Macmillan, London

Peile, C. (1988) 'Research Paradigms in Social Work: From Stalemate to Creative Synthesis', *Social Service Review*, vol. 62, pp. 1–19

Pilalis, J. (1986) 'The Integration of Theory and Practice: A Re-examination of a Paradoxical Expectation', *British Journal of Social Work*, vol. 16, pp. 79–96

Piper, M.H. (1989) 'The Heuristic Paradigm: A Unifying and Comprehensive Approach to Social Work Research', *Smith College Studies in Social Work*, vol. 60, pp. 8–34

Pithouse, A. (1987) *Social Work: The Social Organisation of an Invisible Trade*, Avebury, Aldershot

Rees, S. (1991) *Achieving Power: Practice and Policy in Social Welfare*, Allen & Unwin, Sydney

Rein, M. and White, S. (1981) 'Knowledge for Practice', *Social Service Review*, vol. 55, no. 1, pp. 1–41

Roberts, R. (1990) *Lessons from the Past: Issues for Social Work Theory*, Tavistock/Routledge, London

Rojek, C., Peacock, G. and Collins, S. (1988) *Social Work and Received Ideas*, Routledge, London

Sheldon, B. (1978) 'Theory and Practice in Social Work: A Re-examination of a Tenuous Relationship', *British Journal of Social Work*, vol. 8, no. 1, pp. 1–22

Sibeon, R. (1991) *Towards a New Sociology of Social Work*, Avebury, Aldershot

Smid, G. and Van Krieken, R. (1984) 'Notes on Theory and Practice in Social Work: A Comparative View', *British Journal of Social Work*, vol. 14, pp. 11–22

Smith, D. (1987) *The Everyday World as Problematic*, Northeastern University Press, Boston

Turner, B. (ed.) (1993) *Citizenship and Social Theory*, Sage, London

Weeks, W. (1988) 'De-Professionalisation or a New Approach to Professionalism?', *Australian Social Work*, vol. 41, no. 1, pp. 29–37

Weick, A. (1987) 'Reconceptualizing the Philosophical Perspective of Social Work', *Social Service Review*, vol. 61, pp. 218–30

Wenocur, S. and Reisch, M. (1989) *From Charity to Enterprise: The Development of American Social Work in a Market Economy*, University of Illinois, Urbana and Chicago

Wilding, P. (ed.) (1986), *In Defence of the Welfare State*, Manchester University Press, Manchester

Yeatman, A. (1994) *Postmodern Revisionings of the Political*, Routledge, New York

3 The organisation of social work in the customer culture
Gary Hough

The relationship between individuals and the social structures in which they live has always been at the core of 'social' work. The parallel debate about the roles of action and structure, and particularly about the role of human agency in the production and reproduction of organisational forms, has been at the centre of the study of organisations, and the development of the field of organisational theory. These issues can, of course, be studied from many directions and the study of organisations is characterised by many competing orientations and perspectives, which sometimes complement and sometimes contradict one another (Jones and May 1992: 33).

The organising of human affairs according to metanarratives or grand stories is crucial to postmodern theories, and the history of organisational theory exemplifies this, from the underpinning metaphors of 'the machine' at the beginning of this century to the idea of 'the market' at the end of it:

> Organizations have been imagined in terms of ideal types and
> their deviations, systems and their throughput processes,
> organizations and their contingencies, markets and their structures
> and failures, populations of organizations and their ecologies,
> cultures and their institutionalized myths and ceremonies, as well
> as the realpolitik of power. (Clegg 1990: 2)

In naming these framing ways of describing organisations, and action within them, we should not assume a succession of dominant organisational metanarratives; they live on beside each other (notwithstanding that one or another may be pervasive at particular times).

The rationalist assumptions and prescriptive structures of orthodox organisation theory (the ongoing quest for a 'science' of management) collapsed under the criticisms ushered in by the paradigm revolution (in the 1960s), the development of feminist organisation theory and the rise of critical theory. The rise of postmodernist and deconstructionist approaches over the last two decades has posed a different set of problems; as they have attacked the foundational claims of orthodox Organisation Theory, they have raised the problem not of what should be put in its place, but of whether any such foundational claims about how we should organise (or act, or live) can be made at all. Where critical theorists will see the modernist project as sick but capable of being reconstructed if the good aspects are recovered, postmodernists pronounce its death and view the whole modernist project—founded on the discourse of progress, and premised on more knowledge, more technology, more rationality, more production—as fundamentally wrong. There is no 'thinkable future' to proclaim (Alvesson and Deetz 1996: 194).

Notwithstanding the myriad clashing 'stories' about the essential nature of organisations, there is a very real set of formal institutions in which social and community services are produced, and these have been massively transformed over the last ten to fifteen years in Australia. How we understand the contemporary operation of these institutions, and how we deal with the new problems of enacting and transacting social work within them, is the focus of this chapter.

CRITICAL THEORY, POSTMODERNISM AND ORGANISATION THEORY

In organisation theory, as more generally, a connection between critical theory and postmodern theory is seen by many as necessary. Without integrating some postmodern themes, critical theory becomes unreflective about issues of cultural elitism and power; postmodernism, if it is not to lead to an apolitical or reactionary stance, desperately needs some points of direction and social relevance (Alvesson and Deetz 1996: 211). An all-out attack on the modernist tradition in organisation studies is central to both approaches. This modernist tradition was based on an instrumental approach to people and nature; on scientific and technical knowledge, on predictable results, and on the measurement of productivity. Efficiency has always been its prime value.

There is more than adequate discussion of the core ideas of postmodernism elsewhere in this volume. They were applied to the field of organisation studies by the mid-1980s, and some of the formulations overlapped with the critiques emanating from critical theory from the mid-1970s. Both drew attention to the social, historical and political construction of knowledge, people and social relations (Clegg and Hardy 1996: 16). Both were concerned with unmasking the interests furthered by general managerial control of the organisational world. Not only did they dispute its claims to be apolitical and serving a general interest, but they moved the focus from relatively simple 'on the surface' systems of control to the more subtle and complex control of possibilities fostered through hegemony and then through the control of the mindpower or subjectivities of the workers. Not just class, sex and gender, but social and psychic life, are all defined and re-produced in the enactment of organisational life (Mills and Simmons 1996: 4).

Critical Theory, like postmodernism, embraces a bewildering range of approaches. Broad definitions would include all works taking a critical or radical stance on contemporary society, and having unequal power relations as their prime focus. A narrower definition would apply to the traditions of the Frankfurt School, located by Burrell and Morgan (1979) within a Radical–Humanist paradigm. Some writings from within the action frame of reference, and the actor-network theory (Law 1994), have some of the same concerns, though not all offer the same critique of the status quo.

Critical Theory sought to show the myths that underpinned modernism, but remained ambivalent about the modernist quest. Contemporary society—embodied in science and industrialisation—is seen as having residual positive capacities which have been continually subverted by domination. A broader conception of rationality (to combat the domination of instrumental reasoning), and the inclusion of more groups in decision-making (to combat the attempt to present highly sectional interests as universal) are seen by critical theorists as the way forward. Broadly, such an approach would sit well with most formulations of the over-arching aims of progressive social work over the 1970s and 1980s.

All postmodern approaches will assert the centrality of discourse in structuring, at one and the same time, the world and the person's subjectivity. Social identity is conferred through discourse. Any stabilising forces in this process are more and more stretched, as master narratives or foundational claims or privileged discourses wither under deconstruction. This doesn't mean that they do not have power, or that those who speak them do not increase theirs. In the field of organisations, Ingersoll and Adams (1986: 366) describe a managerial metamyth with three core components:

a   Eventually all work processes can and should be rationalized; that is, broken into their constituent parts and so thoroughly understood that they can be completely controlled.
b   The means for attaining organizational objectives deserves maximum attention, with the result that the objectives quickly become subordinated to the means.
c   Efficiency and predictability are more important than any other consideration.

We can clearly argue that this is just a narrative. But it is one that has massive implications for work/labour (which are not necessarily the same thing), for the nature of the social in organisations, for the implicit assumptions about individuals, the material world, and their relation to it. It may have no more intrinsic persuasive power than any other formulation, but in the contemporary organisational world it has enormous power when large numbers of people are induced or compelled or choose to act in ways that produce and reproduce it.

Beyond naming the myths or narratives that we are prone to seamlessly accept, an attention to discourse will allow us to find the absences and silences in the language of organisations. Mills and Simmons (1996) point out that the famous Hawthorne experiments, which marked the discovery of the informal organisation and the genesis of the human relations school of organisation theory, were centrally organised around issues of gender, but gender was never named in any way in the study. Gender and sexuality are a feature of the workplace, but also of the study of the workplace. 'Rationality' may be assumed to be a universal (however, it is subsequently valued), rather than a male-associated characteristic. The same critiques can be made about radical theories of organisation, or the famous action frame of reference work of Silverman (1970), who has been criticised for accepting male reference points in developing his arguments about the primacy of actors' perceptions (Mills and Simmons 1996: 139). But, even if gender and sexuality do enter the analysis of the workplace, a different set of silences can develop, as different experiences of the intersection of gender, class, sexuality and ethnicity are hidden in the acceptable discourses.

We end up with an expectation of fragmented identities in organisations, with the need for highly specific local narratives about how organisation is continually emergent; where attempts at representation are always partial and one-sided; where subjectivities are shaped as organisation itself is subjectively shaped, produced and consumed.

While postmodernism provides new methods for naming the

processes evident in particular approaches to creating organisation (and clarifying whose interests are served and disserved in any formulation), it shares with critical theory an assumption that social, historical and political forces construct knowledge, social relations and the people who in turn construct them. In summary, we end up with a very different understanding of what 'organisation' is.

THE ORGANISATIONAL CONTEXT OF SOCIAL WORK AT THE END OF THE CENTURY: MANAGED MARKETS

If we 'construct' realities primarily through language, and social structures have no existence outside of the symbols and conventions used by interacting individuals to describe them, does it follow that we have the promise of a world of emancipatory organisations where individuals are freed from the imperatives and restrictions of (the now discredited and demolished) structures? Some writers and theorists proclaim such a world of postmodern organisations—an organisational world of loosely coupled networks where organisations are held together only by transcendental values and the management of meaning itself (Limerick and Cunnington 1993). Paradoxically, while more collectivist work structures and processes are seen as an inevitable outcome of the new order by those who celebrate it, critics are likely to see the same collectivist forms as a promising mode of resistance to the new order—see, for instance, Leonard (1997).

Some theorists view the evidence for 'the' postmodern organisational form as weak and selective (Thompson 1993), and argue that there is most often merely a re-labelling of organic, adhocratic or Post-Fordist organisational forms (Alvesson and Deetz 1996). Others (e.g. Clegg 1990) take a different view, and see the bureaucratic form—which has dominated organisation studies from the outset, as having been comprehensively displaced: from the outside as boundaries break down and blur in clusters, networks and strategic alliances; and from the inside as empowered, flat, flexible structures change the shape of the organisation. Whatever the claims, social workers are likely to have a mixed and contradictory set of experiences of the 1990s workplace.

MANAGERIALISM

In English-speaking reformed economies, our understandings of how we should organise have been propogated by an organisational 'knowledge industry', based around the business schools and management consultancies, and supported by the financial information gatherers—the accountancy profession, stockbrokers, merchant banks and money markets. Although this constellation of actors and interests has been actively aided by the work of the right-wing 'think-tanks', there is no conspiracy. A collection of separate interests coalesce in the broad approach. Somewhat surprisingly, the technologies they propound did not emanate first from industry, but from academia and (atypical sections of) the public sector itself. Managerialism, which should be seen as an ideology, a philosophy, a culture and a set of practices, had, by the end of the 1980s, become the taken-for-granted management style in the Australian public sector.

The principles of managerialism include an emphasis on linking policy analysis (strategic choices) and management planning, with the executive taking responsibility for overall planning and tying outcomes to resources through the control of program budgets. The emphasis is on outputs rather than inputs, the replacement of bureaucratic controls with controls based on goals and objectives laid down at the top of the organisation (and technically implemented further down), the integration of all activities under a guiding corporate plan, and the replacement of rule-based administration with management by objectives. In addition, there is an emphasis on flatter management structures, performance-based appraisal and incentive systems based on merit and tied to transparency in job design and specification, and a reliance on technical expertise rather than value-based practice. A form of accountability is established which indicates a lack of trust in (both) the devolved control of participatory democracy and the procedural integrity of bureaucracy (McTaggart et al. 1991: 123):

> [Managerialism] begins with an imaginary identification where the corporation and management become a unitary entity; its central motif is control; its primary mode of reasoning is cognitive-instrumental; its favoured modality is money; and its favoured site of reproduction is the formal organization. (Deetz 1992: 223)

None of this seems terribly different from what I have characterised above as the modernist tradition in organisation theory. And it isn't. For instance, Buchanan (1995) notes that the:

> emergence of Human Resource Management (HRM) as the dominant ideology for labour management in the 90s does not represent anything particularly new. In many ways it is simply the reworking of old concepts dressed up in [the] contemporary jargon of decentralization of decision making or 'empowerment' of workers. (Buchanan 1995: 65)

Indeed, the overall thrust of HRM practices doesn't seem too different from the 'efficiency engineering' carried out by Henry Ford's 'Sociological Department' in 1914 (Lacey 1987: 161).

How it feels to experience work within the managerialised public sector bureaucracies is familiar to all of us. What is new is the assumption of unity of purpose for the whole organisation (with the denial that groups of workers might have a collective interest—professional or industrial—separate from it), and the imposition of a dominating monoculture within it. In Wilmott's ringing phrase, 'Cultural diversity is dissolved in the acid bath of core corporate values' (Wilmott 1993: 534). I will return to this point later.

Parenthetically, it is important to note the postmodern assumptions about imminence, contestability and fragmentation, which make it no surprise that this dominating discourse of the New Public Management is beginning to break down as it becomes 'the only game in town' and becomes too dominant and too universal for its own good health (Pollitt 1995).

Cutler and Waine (1994), Pollitt (1995) and Ife (1997) have, in different ways, pointed to the continuities managerialism (or, in Pollitt's phrase, 'the New Public Management') displays. These are clear in the embrace of positivist (or sometimes even functionalist) understandings of the social world, and of how performance should be planned, described, implemented and measured. At the same time that 'social engineering' is decried as an approach to social policy, it is supremely embodied in the elaborate processes of classifying consumer groups, targeting and specifying units of service.

But these continuities are confounded by the ideology of the market which coexists (uneasily) in the evolving reformed institutions of the welfare state. In the later waves of managerialism, the centralised and hardly disguised power of managerialism has been harnessed to propogating market modes of operation and exhorting entrepreneurialism. Naming the parts of managerialism can be done comfortably from within a critical theory stance, but in talking about the new cultures of consumerism and the market, we need to incorporate some elements of postmodern approaches, to inform both our analysis and our practice.

THE DISCOURSE OF THE MARKET

The idea of the market is integrally connected to neo-classical economics, and strives for a 'scientific' status through the formal modelling of abstract relationships. At the same time, the market provides a prime contemporary exemplar of the power of language and discourse. The market is an idea—or, in Carrier's words, 'a conception people have about an idealised form of buying and selling' (Carrier 1997: vii). To give it the sort of foundational status that it sometimes seems to demand now (e.g. in transaction cost analysis—see Rowlinson 1997) is to ignore the collective weight of the disciplines of history and anthropology. Totally free markets, independent of (social) institutions and organisations have never existed (Carrier 1997). Yet market forces can now charge organisations and institutions without having to justify themselves for either distorting the market, or for having usurped transactions which belong to the market. The same forces will deny any autonomous existence for the state, beyond providing a safety net in the event of market failure.

The core of the market's claim to pre-eminence lies in the collapse of the bureaucratic model and the impossibility of systems of imperative control prevailing in the face of greater complexity and fragmentation. Organisations are said to have developed to fill the holes caused by market failure. Markets are said to fail when they cannot surmount endemic problems of bounded rationality, complexity, opportunism (or deliberate failure to meet contract conditions) and the problems of dealing efficiently with small numbers. Large institutions (or big, multi-divisional firms) can begin to deal with some of the problems, but because of escalating rigidities and inefficiencies, they too will inevitably fail in the longer term. We are left only with markets again.

Carrier stresses the cultural (and political) power that representations of the market invoke. These representations are based on deep assumptions about human beings who are 'free' to judge their desires, and who should face no constraints beyond those that they voluntarily accept. There can be no definitive moral framework, no general will and no relevance to inquiring about the reasons why people might desire any particular thing (Carrier 1997: 2). If choice becomes the prime moral good, then competition between sellers becomes essential to providing that choice. Moreover, it is assumed that sellers must be centrally concerned with innovation and efficiency, in order to provide choice. This nexus of choice, competition and efficiency means that monopolies among firms or unions, producer groups of any type (including, for instance, those producing 'education' or 'social work') are highly undesirable, as are any forms of subsidy or benefit to firms or individuals.

The decline of manufacturing and the subsequent rise of service and information industries have been attended by a change from the language of capitalism and classes, to 'consumption' and 'the market' (Carrier 1997: 5). Because the market is an idea, it

cannot simply be implemented by governments. Rather, they have
had to settle on specific policies, and to encourage or oblige people
to act in appropriate ways: people must deal with each other in
contract-based ways and they must keep each other at arm's
length. There are many problems with this. Sociological arguments
about the market make the point that people don't always behave
in this way. They are prone to developing ongoing relationships
based on trust and their transactions cumulatively develop a moral
component—in other words, fairness enters. The neo-institutional
approach to studying organisations (Di Maggio and Powell 1983)
makes the obvious point that, in any case, people and
organisations don't always choose rationally. They may copy what
they see as successful choices; they may associate superstitious
factors with particular outcomes (we have Total Quality Management and that explains our success or, conversely, we did not
commit ourselves totally to it, so it did not work); or they may
be punished if they do not adopt the generally validated solutions.

Fundamental criticism of the market lost legitimacy during the
1980s, and even if (systemic) 'gouging, chicanery, inequality and
sheer offensive greed' do seem to go with markets, these are
dismissed as 'distortions' (Carrier 1996: 16). The market has
triumphed, and the setting up of internal markets is always good,
as is treating citizens as customers of government services, or
hiring business consultants to advise on how universities or welfare agencies should be managed.

MANAGED MARKETS

Social workers are likely to be working at the moment in the
worst of all possible organisational worlds—the managed market,
which brings all of the problems of both managerialism and
markets, and few of the claimed benefits of either. Moreover, it
gives us a system riddled with competing imperatives. Ife (1997)
has pointed out that, while managerialism and markets share a
realist view of the world and a deep respect for positivist or
quantitative approaches to describing performance in it, one has
a deep tradition of hierarchy and central control while the other
is close to anarchistic. One specifies the rules that must be
followed; the other exhorts you to be entrepreneurial and 'discover' them.

Total Quality Management provides a good example of a
discourse which seeks to bridge the managerial and market divide.
Systems of quality management characteristically have an elaborate structure of surveillance and control to support 'ideological

exhortation and cultural programming'. TQM seeks to implement a 'technology of governance' where:

> all organizational members are required to submit themselves to a regime of control which empowers them to take direct responsibility for organization action, while at the same time demanding that they exercise complete mastery over their own behaviour in order to deliver the standards of performance which TQM systems expect. (Reed 1995: 53)

The implications for contemporary professional practice are profound. At the same time that professionals are turned into budget holders and inserted into a chain of command, they must operate in entrepreneurial ways in a quasi-market that has been decreed. This quasi-market, unlike 'real' markets, operates within a context of predetermined public policy objectives. The purchaser in the managed market is not the service user, but the professional in a government agency (Cutler and Waine 1994). These workers are to be fully attuned to market signals, but are not free to act in how they respond to them.

ORGANISATIONAL CULTURE AND THE CONSTRUCTION OF SUBJECTIVITIES

I want to use a brief discussion of organisational culture to bring this discussion together.

> At the heart of rationalization stands the greatest contingency of human achievement—material culture, sometimes resisting, sometimes bending, but never discountable, together with the enveloping frame of the state and national institutions, within which organizational forms are fabricated . . . (Clegg 1990: 174)

A burgeoning literature has developed about organisational culture—in the public sector, in the social services and in corporations. Organisational theorists, business managers and public administrators have all become interested in how (organisational) culture is created, sustained, and/or changed. The interest in culture has a long tradition within the sociological study of organisations. Durkheim (1952) noted the decline of traditional patterns of social order, which accompanied the development of organisational societies, as common beliefs and values gave way to more fragmented patterns of belief and practice based on the occupational structure of society. We might discern a transition of at least equal scale as 'modern' belief systems and practices give way in a globalised and increasingly fragmented world.

Shared meaning, shared understanding, and shared sense-making (Weick 1995) are all different ways of describing culture, and a process of reality construction is postulated as allowing people to understand particular events, actions, objects, utterances or situations in distinctive ways (Morgan 1986), and so constitute the shared interpretative schemes which make organisation possible. Despite pervasive attempts in the corporate world to impose a cultural control model, culture cannot be imposed. It can only develop during the course of social interaction and is fabricated principally through discourse and language which frames social processes, images, symbols and rituals. Because there are many competing readings of the organisation, we can expect to find 'a mosaic of organisational realities rather than a uniform corporate culture' (Morgan 1986: 129).

THE CULTURE OF THE CUSTOMER

Du Gay's (1996) recent work is a good example of the type of analysis which can be developed through the judicious use of postmodern and critical theory approaches. He characterises the marketised organisational world as one of identity crises. Such developments as the expansion of services, the globalisation of production and exchange, and the feminisation of the labour force (which supplanted the previous order of large-scale manufacturing, national economies and male breadwinners) have revealed the 'constructed' character of what were seen as 'natural' economic entities. Identity becomes contingent and dislocated as the 'outside' changes. In his examination of the construction of new work identities and the production of different work-based subjects, Du Gay has researched how different categories of persons are 'made up' at work. This process of making up persons is not about work identities or roles: Du Gay is adamant that traditional separations between production and consumption identities—between what is inside and outside the domain of organisational existence—have collapsed. If organisational life is dominated by the language of the consumer culture, then people are encouraged to conflate their identity as consumer and worker. Work is reimagined through the lens of the consumer culture, and the worksite becomes an integral part of the 'lifestyle' of the worker/consumer. In the enterprise culture, everyone is an entrepreneur. The discourse/ideology of excellence posits a win/win situation for the organisation, and for each of the self-seeking and self-creating individuals within it.

Obviously, it is not being assumed that new ways for people to imagine themselves are simply constructed, imposed or determined. Discourse always allows the possibility of its refutation. The subject/object or society/individual constitute each other (Du Gay 1996: 75). The enterprise form crucially sits alongside managerialism because it shares the same propensity to impose one form of logic, one way of imagining the world, or the one 'principle of functioning'. Whatever the enterprise, we are told that the only way to pursue it is through entrepreneurial flexibility. (The paradox is that this same entrepreneurial flexibility is being put in place through the systems of imperative control developed in the newly managerialised public service.) So we have a very muddy field in which organisational actors must 'perform' organisation, and the metaphor of performance, with its connotations of 'presentation' and 'accomplishment', seems particularly apt.

Du Gay has carried out research exploring the processes through which changes in the governance of organisational life have constructed new ways for people to conduct themselves at work. His focus is on how discourses of organisational reform take hold in particular contexts and how 'the dreams and schemes they advocate and articulate are operationalised'; of how employees, in their workaday lives, negotiate the identities which have been constructed for them. This sort of analysis, and the practice of reading and acting in the highly localised but commonly structurated workplace, provides directions for our research, and for our practice. It also will attune us to how our co-workers, and service users, are likely to be experiencing aspects of 'organisation' that we co-produce, and how the organisation is producing our ideas of ourselves.

CONCLUSION

As practitioners, we have to try to make sense of change. Postmodernism is helpful when it exhorts self-reflexiveness and scepticism, but it becomes disabling when it denies us the possibility of making any sense of the changes overwhelming us. It is difficult to take action whilst simultaneously acknowledging that our analyses are contingent and fallible.

We need a theory of organisations that focuses on structure and personality, and on social realities; there are still power holders in the world, and although the self may be fragmentary, our ability to choose the worlds we wish to inhabit is severely constrained. We know that inequality is steadily increasing, and that the job security and conditions of workers are picked off, one by one, as competitive efficiencies lead to greater benefits for us, 'the consumer'.

We may also have to defy postmodern thought in recovering some elements of moral discourse in organisations. There has recently been a renewed interest in the writings of the social work pioneer and settlement house worker, Mary Parker Follett (Harmon 1989; Selber and Austin 1997), who insisted that activity always does more than embody purpose: it evolves it. Moral purpose should become a function of the nature and quality of the social relations through which purposes emerge. This line of argument runs through the action or process approach to organisation theory, and through the critical theory school (Harmon 1989).

We need to declaim the postmodern tenet about the celebration of difference, the affirmation of different subjectivities and the need for the preservation and redevelopment of subcultures within organisations.

We can be more alert to the stories about organisation that we tell ourselves, and that we tell to others. There are symbolic, emotional and political aspects of organising and, although these have always been ignored—or at best marginalised—by the (modernist) scientific rationality which still dominates management theory and practice (Chia 1996), we can tell localised stories which have some theoretical power, without totalising them.

It may be helpful for workers to conceptualise their work less in terms of fixed roles and tasks, and more as entrepreneurial projects; however, the language we use to frame these projects, for ourselves and others, is crucial. Mainstream discourses can be appropriated and used strategically. Critical postmodernism alerts us to the potential for local patterns of organising to stabilise and reproduce themselves.

Organisations are always in a state of becoming, and social workers, in their everyday practice and through their micro-activities, can make the world more amenable to human intervention and the fulfilment of social projects.

REFERENCES

Alvesson, M. and Deetz, S. (1996) 'Critical Theory and Postmodernism', in S. Clegg, R. Stewart, C. Hardy and W. Nord (eds), *Handbook of Organization Studies*, Sage, London, pp. 191–217
Buchanan, J. (1995) 'Managing Labour in the 1990s', in S. Rees and G. Rodley (eds), *The Human Costs of Managerialism*, Pluto Press, Sydney

Burrell, G. and Morgan, G. (1979) *Sociological Paradigms and Organizational Analysis*, Heinemann, London

Carrier, J. (ed.) (1997) *Meanings of the Market*, Berg Publishers, Oxford

Chia, R. (1996) 'Towards a Postmodern Science of Organization' *Organization*, vol. 3, no. 1, pp. 31–59

Clegg, S. (1990) *Modern Organizations: Organization Studies in the Postmodern World*, Sage, London

Clegg, S. and Hardy, C. (1996) 'Organizations, Organization and Organizing', in S. Clegg, C. Hardy and W. Nord (eds), *Hardbook of Organization Studies*, Sage, London

Cutler, T. and Waine, B. (1994) *The Politics of Managerialism*, Berg Publishers, Oxford

Du Gay, P. (1996) *Consumption and Identity at Work*, Sage, London

Durkheim, E. (1952) *Suicide*, Routledge, London

Harmon, M. (1989) ' "Decision" and "action" as contrasting perspectives in organization theory', *Public Administration Review*, March/April, pp. 144–51

Hassard, J. and Parker, M. (eds) (1993) *Postmodernism and Organizations*, Sage, London

Ife, J. (1997) *Rethinking Social Work*, Longman, Melbourne

Ingersoll, V. and Adams, G. (1986) 'Beyond Organizational Boundaries: Exploring the Managerial Metamyth', *Administration and Society*, 18, pp. 360–81

Jones, A. and May J. (1992) *Working in Human Service Organizations*, Longman Cheshire, Melbourne

Lacey, R. (1987) *Ford*, Pan Books, London

Law, J. (1994) *Organizing Modernity*, Blackwell, Oxford

Leonard, P. (1997) *Postmodern Welfare*, Sage, London

Limerick, D. and Cunnington, B. (1993) *Managing the New Organization*, Business and Professional Publishing, Sydney

McTaggart, R., Caulley, D. and Kemmis, S. (1991) 'Evaluation Traditions in Australia', *Evaluation and Program Planning*, no. 14, pp. 123–30

Mills, A. and Simmons, T. (1996) *Reading Organization Theory*, Garamond Press, Toronto

Morgan, G. (1986) *Images of Organization*, Sage, Beverly Hills, California

Newton, T. (1996) 'Postmodernism and Action', *Organization*, vol. 3, no. 1, pp. 7–29

Pollitt, C. (1995) 'Justification by Works or by Faith? Evaluating the New Public Management', *Evaluation*, vol. 1, no. 2, pp. 133–54

Reed, M. (1995) 'Managing Quality in Organizational Politics: TQM as a Governmental Technology', in I. Kirkpatrick and M. Martinez Lucio (eds), *The Politics of Quality in the Public Sector*, Routledge, London

—— (1996) 'Organizational Theorizing: A Historically Contested Terrain' in S. Clegg, R. Stewart, C. Hardy and W. Nord (eds), *Handbook of Organization Studies*, Sage, London

Rowlinson, M. (1997) *Organizations and Institutions*, Macmillan Press Ltd, Hampshire

Selber, K. and Austin, D. (1997) 'Mary Parker Follett: Epilogue to or Return of a Social Work Management Pioneer', *Administration in Social Work*, vol. 21, no. 1, pp. 1–15

Silverman, D. (1970) *The Theory of Organizations*, Heinemann Educational Books, London

Thompson, P. (1993) 'Post-Modernism: Fatal Distraction', in J. Hassard and M. Pasher (eds), *Postmodernism and Organizations*, Sage, London

Weick, K. (1995) *Sensemaking in Organizations*, Sage, Thousand Oaks, Cal.

Wilmott, H. (1993) 'Strength is Ignorance, Slavery is Freedom: Managing Culture in Modern Organizations', *Journal of Management Studies*, vol. 30, no. 4, pp. 515–52

PART II
Dealing with diversity and difference

4 Social work ethics: Embracing diversity? Linda Briskman and Carolyn Noble

INTRODUCTION

This chapter presents our reflections arising from practice, research and teaching which led us to question the relevance of
universal codes of ethics in light of the rapid theoretical developments that have occurred in social work over the last 25 years.
In particular, our concern was to evaluate if (or how) professional
codes of ethics, like the current Australian Association of Social
Work (AASW) code, engaged with progressive politics, a dominant
discourse of this period. This progressive view emphasised power
relations associated with class, gender, age, ability, sexuality and
ethnicity.

This view, in turn, informed an anti-discriminatory practice
integrating individual and structural perspectives in an empowering practice mode (Moreau 1979; Langan and Day 1992; Fook
1993; Mullaly 1997). This led to an exploration of codes of ethics
in other comparable countries and a confrontation, for us, with
the individualistic politics of liberal thought, characteristic of the
AASW code, that characterised their underlining philosophical
perspective (see Noble and Briskman 1996a, 1996b). We found
that these codes emphasised individual choice, minimising structural disadvantage and social dependency.

We turned to postmodernism as a means to critique the issues
we found problematic. This is consistent with a developing critique
of universalising approaches which has arisen in tandem with the
emergence of postmodern perspectives in social work generally
(Howe 1994; Leonard 1994, 1997). This analysis is part of a
journey we have taken, over the last four years, to try to formulate
a more relevant code or moral framework for the profession, a
journey fraught with ideological and political tensions.

A major difficulty in our quest has been having to grapple with the application of the postmodern perspective in the codification of practice. We agree with Bauman (1993: 245), who suggests: 'the postmodern perspective offers more wisdom; [but] the postmodern setting makes acting on that wisdom more difficult'. Yet, as social workers, we contend that we need to find pathways to act on that wisdom and apply the lessons of the postmodern paradigm to practice. It is our contention that the notion of an all-encompassing code of ethics which emphasises universality, inclusiveness and conventional conceptualisations of community in fact mutes the diverse interests and plurality of voices characteristics of modern pluralist societies. However, we also concur with Fawcett and Featherstone (1996: 211), who assert their wish to dissociate themselves from a postmodern approach which seems to 'condemn everything and propose nothing'—what we have coined 'theory without a cause'.

With these tensions in mind, we have engaged in a process of research and dialogue in order to explore a framework for the articulation of difference and acceptance of socio-cultural diversity in which diverse voices, particularly those normally excluded from public debate, have an equal right to be included in any code of ethics. How to turn these theoretical ideals into practice, as Lister (1997) notes, is a critical question and one that has provided us with a launching pad for our inquiry.

THE EMERGENCE OF CODES OF ETHICS

Traditionally, codes of ethics have been one of the defining aspects of a profession (Banks 1995). Reasons identified for the emergence of codes of ethics in professions include the following: as a contribution to the professional status of an occupation; to establish and maintain professional identity; to guide practitioners about how to act; and to protect users from malpractice or abuse (Banks 1995: 89). At a broader level, codes consisting of statements of values or general moral principles that can be accepted by all members of the profession are a means for applying idealistic principles guiding professional behaviour to specific professional activities. Siggins (1996: 55) sees the development of ethics and codes of practice in recent times—not only in the professions but in business, industry and social services—as a response to the successful growth of consumer movements and their demand for accountability to the public interest.

Preston (1996: 8) regards the re-emergence of concerns with ethics as a serious attempt by some sections of the professions to

engage in reflective, critical and transformative debate with changing social and technological conditions aimed at benefiting those
most disadvantaged in those contexts. Such an approach recognises that ethical behaviour takes place within a complex
interaction of social forces and vested interests. Gilligan (1982)
and Porter (1991) identify differing moral reasoning between men
and women. Rossiter et al. (1996) call into question the individualistic prescriptions for ethics found in the mainstream
professional literature, and in the bureaucratic structure of human
service organisations where ethical decision-making frequently
takes place. They argue for a model of intersubjectivity to replace
the individual prescriptions that separate workers from constructive and reflective dialogue (Rossiter et al. 1996: 48).

RETHINKING CODES OF ETHICS

Our examination of the codes of a number of countries, including
Canada and the United States, supported our concerns about the
critical lag between progressive theory and ethics (Noble and
Briskman 1996b). Our findings support Rossiter et al.'s (1996)
concerns, emerging from their research into the Canadian code,
as 'rule bound, distant, prescriptive that denied social dependence
and structural influences' (1996: 46). In the main, we found that
these codes incorporated, at best, global assumptions based on
general notions of social justice, elimination of discrimination and
self-determination. It is implicit in the Australian Code (1990) that
moral and ethical evaluation, in relation to practice issues, implies
a universality of ethical claims. These can be perceived and
measured by an implied concept of logic and reason, as well as a
notion of agency, which discusses all clients and all social workers
as having common concerns and occupying the same political
positions in society (Noble and Briskman 1996a: 58).

Rhodes (1986) advances concerns about the application of
justice principles within the US (NASW) Code of Ethics, arguing
that there is no general agreement on such fundamental concepts.
She states (1986: 13) that the 'New Right's' conception of justice
differs from that of the 'liberals' which differs again from 'socialist' conceptions. By not spelling out the nature of justice, social
workers cannot be expected to understand the form of their
responsibility or the outcome they are working towards.

As social work associations which are members of the International Federation of Social Workers (IFSW) are required to write
a code consistent with the IFSW Code of Ethics (Gaha 1996: 101),
it is perhaps not surprising that many aspects of social work codes

in different countries are similar. We found, in our research, that the codes are universally informed by, and place high value on, individualism, independence and homogeneity of the client characterised by a liberal democratic philosophy (Noble and Briskman 1996b). This position is in direct contrast to the postmodernist notion of differently positioned subjects where differently positioned social actors (women, gay men, lesbians, indigenous people, migrants and children) cannot be incorporated into a collective struggle. Nor can they be assumed to share a unified value system and moral perspective which are represented in universalist and uniform codes.

Our concern that social work, in the main, continues to look at 'one approach fits all' attracted us to a postmodern analysis of social work ethics in line with Williams (1996: 69), who argues for a theoretical development which takes account of what she defines as the 'conceptual markers' of postmodernist thinking—particularism, difference, relativism, contingency, fragmentation, (de)construction—and works out their relationship to the 'modernist precursors' of universalism, commonality, truth, pattern, structure, essentialism and determinism.

SHOULD A CODE OF ETHICS EXIST?

The quest for us—to link postmodern perspectives and the politics of difference with the search for a new Australian code of ethics—has led us to ask whether a code should exist at all. And, if so, how can such a code give full recognition to differently positioned groups or individuals? The literature presents a range of views on these questions.

Hugman and Smith (1995) posit that, as ethical issues are at the heart of the social work profession, we must expect such codes to be constantly disputed and evolving for a profession to be robust, relevant and living. Bauman (1993) goes so far to suggest that ethics themselves are 'denigrated or derided as one of the typically modern constraints now broken and destined for the dustbin of history' (1993: 2). He cites examples of writers such as Lipvetsky, who suggests that we have entered an era where our conduct has been freed from the last vestiges of oppressive infinite duties, commandments and absolute obligations (in Bauman 1993: 2). Does his argument mean that professional codes of ethics are no longer relevant? Bauman (1993) is ambivalent, arguing that the novelty of the postmodern approach to ethics consists not of the abandoning of modern moral concerns but of the rejection of the 'typically modern ways' of going about moral problems that respond to moral challenges with 'coercive normative regulation in political practice, and the philosophical search for absolutes, universals and foundations in theory' (1993: 3–4).

Banks (1995) raises doubts as to whether codes of ethics can assume a consensus of values, both within the professions and amongst their public. The kind of ethical issues to be considered at both practice and policy levels, where policies are framed for strangers and where there is a diverse and complex range of responses as a result, are different from the kind of ethical considerations operating at the level of intervention where a worker is responding to a particular individual in a particular relationship (Jordan 1995: 53). Additionally, how can a reformulated code address the issue raised by a respondent in our research, who commented on the lack of interest of many social workers in human rights issues (Noble and Briskman 1998a)? How can it help us respond to Amnesty International (1997) reports about the plight of asylum seekers in Australia, to debates about Aboriginal land rights and to the decline in welfare provision in Australia, the United Kingdom and the United States? Riley (1996), in discussing a specific case scenario as a hospital social worker, documented how 'modernist' theories of social work did not allow her to deal adequately with the scope of responses she faced when dealing with a mother who murdered her child. She found that calling on the modernist theoretical perspectives did not deal with the contradictions facing her in trying to provide explanations for the inconsistencies and concerns she experienced when dealing with this complex and extraordinary event (1996: 37).

The social justice provisions of the Australian Code do not extend to political advocacy. In the light of current market-driven organisational and political agendas—although the current Australian code supports endeavours to 'effect change' (Section 4.3)—there is not, as De Maria (1997) points out, overt support in the existing code for activist activities. Yet some writers dispute the need for a code to provide all the answers. For example, Loewenberg and Dolgoff (1992: 33) would argue that the generalised nature of the code permits adjustment to the unique features of each situation.

Our research with academics teaching ethics in progressive Schools of Social Work in Melbourne and Sydney indicated unanimous support for a general code which is flexible in its interpretation. At the same time the academics were critical of it for not going far enough in defining what notions of social justice should inform practice and its lack of specific commitment to progressive politics (Noble and Briskman 1998b). Some unresolved perils remain, however, even in accepting the possibility of reframing a code in which there is recognition of the reality of socio-cultural and political diversity. Using the example of 'woman', Williams (1996: 70) highlights the difficulties emerging as a result of emphasising difference—for example, by asking such questions as whether all differences are the same, whether all differences are to be celebrated, and whether, if we go on recognising differences within differences, we are left with any meaningful category of 'woman'. And where does this position leave notions of commonality, solidarity and consensus for people who may share similarities in their differences? The danger of an unrestrained emphasis on difference, argues Leonard (1997: 165), is that 'it will lead to cultural exclusiveness, restricted identities or intense individualism'.

Leonard (1997) discusses the need to navigate our way through the moral obligations relating to both difference and solidarity. He argues that the moral responsibility to act upon the mutual interdependence of human subjects should not be seen as a problem. Further, he claims, recognition of mutual interdependence is at the core of our subjectivity and is a 'precondition for any effective ideological counter-move to the dominant, narcissistic individualism of the culture of late capitalism' (1997: 164). Flax (1990: 233) notes that the questions remain of how to resolve conflict among competing voices, to ensure that everyone has a chance to speak, and how to ensure that each voice counts equally. Given that the provision of a code appears to be a non-negotiable requirement of professional activity, the solution may rest with a reformulated code, and one which takes into account and champions the multitude of emerging concerns.

If we accept the impossibility of now finding 'one voice' in which to represent difference and if we use what Yeatman (1994) refers to as a politics of difference, where dialogical discussion accepts conflict and confrontation in working towards a negotiated settlement (1994: 89), then it may be possible to have a Code of Ethics that reflects diversity and difference within a multicultural polity. The appeal of a postmodern ethics, according to Leonard (1997: 151), is that it asserts a responsibility to otherness, to those people who have no control over their lives—who have been reduced to objects and are acted upon by 'those with knowledge'. Lister (1997) stresses the importance of emphasising a commitment to dialogue in which participants remain rooted in their own identities and values, while at the same time are willing to shift views in dialogue with those who have other identities and values. A reformulated code would take these negotiated voices as a starting point.

The challenge then remains as to what might exist if social work codes of ethics were based on postmodernist concepts of celebrating and accepting diversity, difference and multiplicity. In the dialogue in which such a framework might occur, it would be essential to ensure a creative tension between these concepts. For this exploration, we turned for some guidelines to both the socio-economic and cultural contexts in which social work currently operates and to our research with practitioners working in areas of social work where diversity was evident, and academics teaching ethics in progressive Schools of Social Work. We also offer the example of New Zealand, where the professional association has attempted to incorporate difference in the reframing of its social work code.

WHAT WOULD A REFORMULATED CODE INCLUDE?

Williams (1996: 74), in the British context, has pointed out that the managerialist notion of diversity and difference has entered welfare discourses through legislation and policy. This is the same in other contexts. For example, in Australia for a number of years, we have seen policy documents that 'target' certain groups labelled as disadvantaged, including women, indigenous groups, people from non-English speaking backgrounds and rural dwellers. To some extent, this trend reflects the state's recognition of the rights of categories smaller than the nation—including ethnic, territorial, religious, gender and sexual-policy based rights—to moral specificity and self-determination—or rather, to allow such a self-determination to happen by default rather than design (Bauman 1993: 45).

Our own research with small groups of social work practitioners in Sydney and Melbourne, all of whom self-identified as coming from a critical, radical or feminist perspective, highlighted that indeed it was difficult to apply the global assumptions in the Australian Association of Social Work Code to specific situations (Noble and Briskman 1998a). Some of those specific situations referred to by practitioners included working with refugees, people from non-English speaking backgrounds, survivors of sexual assault and those suffering from HIV/AIDS. Criticisms from practitioners included that the code was not adequate in addressing issues of gender, sexuality, ethnicity, race, disability, age and class (Noble and Briskman 1998a). Others criticised the middle-class and Western notions and Anglo-Celtic institutions on which the code was seen to be based, through its limited reflection of other world views and diversity of practice. One participant, in particular, referred to this lack of understanding as 'cultural imperialism' (Noble and Briskman 1998a). Most said that they rarely referred to the code in their practice.

Instead, users are increasingly demanding that their services be delivered in terms of their own values, not those of the profession. In Australia, we have observed that a number of agencies are framing codes of ethics specific to their client-base and service delivery—for example, sexual assault centres and indigenous organisations. The Centre Against Sexual Assault (CASA) in Melbourne, for example, has developed its own code of ethics based on the philosophy of that organisation, which incorporates—among other things—components on recognition of sexual assault as a violation of human rights and as a consquencer and reinforcer of the power disparity between men and women (CASA House n.d.).

Developing constituency-based codes or groups is another possible solution. Liggens et al. (1995) have developed an inclusive approach to affirming diversity to sexuality education in schools. This inclusive approach aims to create a social climate where lesbian, gay and bisexual people are accepted and supported and can live without fear of discrimination (1995: 20). Endeavours have also been made to develop ethical guidelines for feminist therapists (Siegal and Larson 1990), which emphasise cultural diversities and oppression as well as power differentials. Regardless of the best way to move forward, Rossiter et al. (1996) argue for the need for practitioners to 'find a space' where uncertainty is tolerated and where 'just norms' are developed within the process of unconstrained speech by all persons affected by the norm in question. We assume that to include clients in these discussions would extend this democratisation to all concerned and lead the way forward to incorporate a diversity of voices in the framing of constituency-based ethical concerns.

There is growing practice evidence which suggests some attempts to challenge and redress the universalising approach to every situation. Freedman and Stark (1991) discuss how, in partnership with indigenous communities in the Mallee region of Victoria, they reframed the concept of foster care to challenge and ultimately change the way the principles behind state government and community agency standards on foster care programs reflected dominant white interests in parenting and, more particularly, mothering. By adopting an 'extended care' model of substitute parenting, the Mallee example highlighted the particularity of the cultural context. This is consistent with the argument proposed by Flax (1990: 176) that there cannot be a uniform experience and discourse of mothering as the practices of mothering vary by race. In human service work, as a further example, advocates of a multicultural service incorporate cultural/ethnic difference 'orientated to the substantive particularity of individual and group needs, where this orientation is a function of ongoing dialogue between service users and service deliverers' (Yeatman 1994: 86). Additionally, Aboriginal groups in Australia are directly contesting their oppression by revaluing and positively acclaiming what makes them different in relation to the dominant norm. This is particularly evident in the quest for land rights.

In addition to these practice examples, there is some evidence of attempts to reframe codes of ethics that specifically represent the diversity of interests and voices that are acknowledged in pluralist societies. For us, the New Zealand code stood out as an example. Reformulated in 1993, the New Zealand Association of Social Workers (NZASW) Code of Ethics attempts to accommodate difference and diversity in an emancipatory and social justice sense which, in turn, offers some direction for change. Section C of this code, the Bicultural Code of Practice of the NZASW, gives recognition that power over resources and decision-making is at present held by Pakeha and acknowledges that: 'Bicultural practice must occur at a structural as well as an individual level to achieve social justice for the Maori' (NZASW 1993). Thus the NZASW, in accommodating the positional difference of the Maori, illustrates the significance of the Maori position in relation to the Pakeha position and shows how a negotiated compromise between irresolvably different concepts of social justice can be achieved without the stronger imposing its will on the weaker (Noble and Briskman 1996a: 7). In contrast to the New Zealand code, the Australian code does not address indigenous concerns. Butler (1997: 7) believes that the Australian social work profession could "take a leaf" from the New Zealand code by consulting with indigenous organisations about the development of a Bicultural Code of Practice'. Similarly, Gaha (1996: 103) refers to one of the omissions of the current Australian code as not taking into account indigenous perspectives on ethical positions. We would also argue that this should be true for women, gay men and lesbians, children, cultural communities and the differently abled.

Our research with academics teaching ethics in progressive Schools of Social Work in Melbourne and Sydney, in commenting on what a revised code might include, reinforced the notion of a dialogical process which involves consulting with clients about what might be in their interests (Noble and Briskman 1998b). Using a community development model, clients could come together and define what social work is and what it should be, giving voices to those marginalised by the current code's emphasis on professional standards and the more conservative, liberal perspective. Additionally, there was agreement that a revised code

> needs to make strong proactive statements about political actions, social change using advocacy as an active part of their work . . . it needs [also] to include issues around power, gender, NESB and politics and engage more critically in systematic abuse perpetrated by social work as a profession and as individuals. (Noble and Briskman 1998b)

RETHINKING THE PROJECT

Postmodernity questions the previous way social work categorised its constituent groupings. Taking a postmodern perspective, it is no longer possible to make assumptions about, for example, all women, all indigenous peoples, all lesbians and gay men, all children, all rural dwellers, and all ethnic and religious minorities. We recognise that many practising social workers would deny working on 'universalist' assumptions in respect to the above 'categories' and would hail individual difference as paramount to their practice methods. Yet, in our view, theoretical concepts, policy assumptions and funding constraints under which such workers operate do not reflect such difference and continue to order individuals into groupings under which they are provided with services. Our research has highlighted the dilemmas for one universalising code of ethics for different agency settings and client focus. Actions may be right in one sense and wrong in another. Thus, in the reality of practice, the substantive particularity of individual and group needs (Yeatman 1994: 86) is side-stepped. The acceptance of otherness, an acknowledgment and celebration of diversity, and recognition that there is no general position of dominance are the foundations from which a reformulated code would start.

However, the acknowledgment of the particularities of individuals and groups poses further dilemmas for the politics of social work. Ethical guidelines have traditionally formed the basis of collective group censure as well as outlining collective commitment to values, norms and moral behaviour that encompasses individual and group good. In claiming a universality, it was possible to work towards challenging large-scale social injustices and to claim a solidarity working towards social and political change. As Leonard (1997) argues, the focusing on the different, the local, the specific need could, in turn, lead to different political limitations than those discussed with modernity. This may yet be true. However, the introduction of cultural, gender, ability and sexual relevance negotiated with a moral responsibility to otherness opens up other possibilities for mutual expression and acceptance of difference yet to be experienced. It must be remembered that these negotiations are always ongoing and are therefore provisional (Yeatman 1994), making interaction, negotiation, compromise and settlement a condition of the process, thus preventing any one privileged position from emerging as dominant.

CONCLUSION

Despite the intensities of this debate, we remain convinced that a reformulated code, in light of the postmodernist concern for diversity and otherness, is a crucial project. We also acknowledge that these theoretical leads now need a translation into practice, specifically into codes of ethics which reach beyond tokenism in the areas of diversity, identity, social justice and celebration of difference. Postmodernism demands space for a multitude of subjectivities for those previously excluded and rendered invisible (Leonard 1997: 157). In this chapter we have taken the lead in developing principles from which a reformulated code might emerge. Following the New Zealand example, a bicultural code would address cultural difference. In organisations, agency-based and/or constituency-based codes would give acknowledgment and voice to different actors and give a positive validation to difference. Practice partnerships that included ongoing dialogue between service users and service providers would address power imbalances and generate a negotiated compromise between differing perspectives. Using a community development model, it might be possible to include the many services users in reframing a code that speaks to their perception of what social work is about and how their many realities can be included. Langan and Day (1992) remind us that theoretical developments in social work do not just represent another addition to ideas, but a fundamental challenge to norms and values, to the whole process of thinking in moral reasoning which has held sway for centuries. Hugman and Smith (1995: 6) alert us to the challenge of 'whether social work should hold to its modernist roots or seize the postmodernist moment and be remoulded ethically according to context and subject'. These are indeed major issues confronting the framers of codes as we enter the new millennium.

RERERENCES

Amnesty International (1997) *Ethnicity & Nationality: Refugees in Asia*
Australian Association of Social Workers (1990) *Code of Ethics*
Banks, S. (1995) *Ethics and Values in Social Work*, Macmillan, London
Bauman, Z. (1993) *Postmodern Ethics*, Blackwell, Oxford
Butler, B. (1997) 'Outcomes Influencing Social Work: The Policies of the
    Removal of Aboriginal Children and its Impact on Social Work', address
    to 25th Australian Association of Social Work National Conference,
    Canberra, September
Canadian Association of Social Workers (1983) *Code of Ethics*
Centre Against Sexual Assault, undated, *Code of Ethics*, Melbourne
De Maria, W. (1997) 'Flapping on Clipped Wings: Social Work Ethics in
    the Age of Activism', *Australian Social Work*, vol. 50, no. 4, pp. 3–19
Fawcett, B. and Featherstone, B. (1996) 'Issues of Evaluation in Social Work
    Education in a Postmodern Era', in *Participation in Change—Social
    Work Profession in Social Development, Proceedings of Joint World
    Congress of IFSW and IASSW,* Hong Kong, pp. 210–12
Flax, J. (1990) *Thinking Fragments: Psychoanalysis, Feminism and
    Postmodernism in the Contemporary West,* University of California
    Press, Berkeley
Fook, J. (1993) *Radical Casework: A Theory of Practice,* Allen & Unwin,
    Sydney
Freedman, L. and Stark, L. (1991) 'When the White System Doesn't Fit', in
    R. Batten, W. Weeks and J. Wilson (eds), *Issues Facing Australian
    Families: Human Services Respond,* Longman, Melbourne
Gaha, J. (1996), 'A Professional Code of Ethics—An Imperfect Regulator',
    *Proceedings of the Third Annual Conference of the Australian Associ-
    ation for Professional and Applied Ethics,* Wagga Wagga, October
Gilligan, C. (1982) *In a Different Voice: Psychological Theory and Women's
    Development,* Harvard University Press, Mass.
Howe, D. (1994) 'Modernity, Postmodernity and Social Work', *British
    Journal of Social Work*, vol. 24, no. 5, pp. 513–32
Hugman, R. and Smith, D. (1995) *Ethical Issues in Social Work,* Routledge,
    London
Jordan, T. (1995) 'Applied Ethics and Action Research Methods', *Proceed-
    ings of the Second Annual Conference of the Australian Association of
    Professional and Applied Ethics,* Brisbane, September
Langan, M. and Day, L. (eds) (1992) *Women, Oppression and Social Work:
    Issues in Anti-Discriminatory Practice,* Routledge, London
Leonard, P. (1994) 'Knowledge/Power and Postmodernism, Implications for
    the Practice of a Critical Social Work Education', *Canadian Social Work
    Review*, vol. 11, no. 1, winter, pp. 11–26
Leonard, P. (1997) *Postmodern Welfare: Reconstructing an Emancipatory
    Project,* Sage, London
Liggens, S., Wille, A., Hawthorne, A. and Rampton, L. (1995) *Affirming*

Diversity: An Educational Resource on Gay, Lesbian and Bisexual Orientations, New Zealand Family Planning Association, Auckland

Lister, R. (1997) *Citizenship: Feminist Perspectives*, Macmillan, London

Loewenburg, F.M. and Dolgoff, R. (1992) *Ethical Decisions for Social Work*, F.E. Peacock Publishers, Itasca

Moreau, M. (1979) 'A Structural Approach to Social Work Practice', *Canadian Journal of Social Work Education*, vol. 5, no. 1, pp. 78–94

Mullaly, R. (1997) *Structural Social Work: Ideology, Theory and Practice*, Oxford University Press, Toronto

National Association of Social Workers (1980) *Code of Ethics*

New Zealand Association of Social Workers (1993) *Code of Ethics*

Noble, C. and Briskman, L. (1996a) 'Social Work Ethics: Is Moral Consensus Possible?', *Women in Welfare Education Journal*, no. 2, July, pp. 53–68

——(1996b) 'Social Work Ethics: The Challenge to Moral Consensus, *Social Work Review* (New Zealand), September, vol. viii, no. 3, pp. 2–9

——(1998a forthcoming) 'Workable Ethics: Social Work and Progressive Practice', *Australian Social Work*

——(1998b) 'Social Work Ethics: Dissonance between Theory and Values', paper presented to the Joint World Conference of the IFSW and IASSW, Jerusalem, July

Porter, E. (1991) *Women and Moral Identity*, Allen & Unwin, Sydney

Preston, N. (1996) *Understanding Ethics*, The Federation Press, Sydney

Rhodes, M.L. (1992) 'Social Work Challenges: The Boundaries of Ethics', *Families in Society*, January, pp. 40–47

Rossiter, A., Prilleltensky, I. and Bowers, R.W. (1996) 'Learning from Broken Rules: Individualism, Organisation and Ethics', in *Participation in Change—Social Work Profession in Social Development, Proceedings of Joint World Congress of IFSW and IASSW*, Hong Kong, pp. 46–49

Riley, A. (1996) 'Murder and Social Work', *Australian Social Work*, vol. 49, no. 2, June, pp. 37–43

Siegal, R.J. and Larson, C.C. (1990) 'The Ethics of Power Differentials', in H. Leuman and N. Porter (eds), *Feminist Ethics in Psychotherapy*, Springer, New York

Siggins, I. (1996) 'Professional Codes: Some Historical Antecedents', in M. Coady and S. Bloch (eds), *Codes of Ethics and the Professions*, Melbourne University Press, Melbourne

Williams, F. (1996) 'Postmodernism, Feminism and the Question of Difference', in N. Parton (ed.), *Social Theory, Social Change and Social Work*, Routledge, London

Yeatman, A. (1994) *Postmodern Revisionings of the Political*, Routledge, New York

5 Challenging victimisation in practice with young women
Karen Crinall

We live in an age of referral mechanisms which have helped diffuse professional responsibilities towards young women . . . a fundamental question exists—at what point do we, as service providers, become abusers . . .? (Kerry Walker, November 1991)

INTRODUCTION

This chapter examines how poststructural feminist theory informs practice with young women experiencing multiple disadvantages: homelessness; gender, race and age discrimination; physical, emotional and sexual violence; poverty and family disconnection. While these young women do not constitute an homogeneous group, they do share experiences of personal and systemic victimisation. At the same time, many of these young women engage in practices and behaviours that display active resistance to becoming victims. This chapter explores some paradoxes of the process of victimisation and makes suggestions as to how practice based on poststructural analysis might be of use in working with young women to develop effective challenges to the operation of victimising processes.

During a period of fourteen years, between 1979 and 1993, I had the privilege of working in a range of settings, including a women's refuge, cottage-homes, youth refuges and a crisis centre with young women experiencing homelessness. For the latter part of that time, I was engaged in examining what feminism may have to offer workers practising with these young women. The combination of social welfare practice and academic inquiry provided opportunity for some fruitful observation and reflection on gender and power in state-funded residential settings. Deriving from these experiences, this chapter seeks to offer some reflections, observations and suggestions on how an emerging feminist discourse informed by poststructural theory might contribute to welfare practice with young women like these.

I found that reframing the meanings attached to young women's homelessness within a feminist poststructural framework broadened possibilities for a more emancipatory practice. Through this process, my expectations, based on established feminist practice frameworks of how young women should present and behave, were challenged.

I wish to stress that this discussion does not represent a backlash directed at the feminist movement or its immense achievements. My concern is that feminist welfare workers extend and pursue social work's tradition of self-reflexivity. As Kerry Walker (1991) reminds us, we must be prepared to examine and address how our practice might reinforce or contribute to exploitative systems of power and processes of victimisation when providing services for young women.

YOUNG WOMEN'S EXPERIENCES OF HOMELESSNESS

Without having been a homeless person, it is not possible to know how homelessness feels. However, it is important that we attempt to achieve some sense of the ontological experience of homelessness for young women. This section is therefore concerned with establishing some of the conditions and circumstances young women face while homeless.

Young women experiencing homelessness confront a range of oppressions. Their disadvantage is multi-layered: they do not have access to safe, secure accommodation; they are poor; if their education is not already severed, they struggle to maintain schooling (Human Rights and Equal Opportunity Commission 1989); and they are female. In many instances, these young women have become disconnected from significant family members able to care for, support and nurture them. This is both a reason for and result of their homelessness. Many have experienced what the *Children and Young Person's Act* 1989 (Vic) describes as '*significant* harm from abuse and/or neglect, variously; physical, psychological, emotional and sexual' (Hirst 1989; Human Rights and Equal Opportunity Commission 1989; Davis 1992). Even so, these young women do not constitute a group or subculture because of their homelessness. Their heterogeneity is evidenced by diverse cultural, class, religious, race and family backgrounds. They do, however, share gendered experiences deriving from social and cultural constructions of masculinity and femininity and the unequal power relationships between men and women. These gendered experiences are connected also to the beliefs and behaviours of family, peers, educational institutions, social networks, the state and the services and agencies funded to address homelessness.

Sexual assault, abuse and harassment are ever-present themes in these young women's lives. Youth workers and welfare agencies suggest that approximately 90 per cent of homeless young women are escaping from sexual and physical abuse (Salvation Army 1993). Observations from my own experience put the figure at about 80 per cent. If the reason for exiting home is not abuse, inevitably young women face sexual harassment often leading to assault and/or abuse in accommodation facilities or short-term living arrangements (Hirst 1989; Alder and Sandor 1989; Davis 1992). The Salvation Army's 'Forced Exit' report found that young women often avoided emergency accommodation for fear of harassment and abuse (Hirst 1989). There is little hope of finding security, support and adequate nurture in out-of-home care.

The state's inadequacy and neglect as a parent is well documented. In 1989, the Human Rights and Equal Opportunity Commission reported:

> the state authorities charged with their [young people in care] protection, and support seriously failed in their duties. The results inflicted on some children because of such official neglect have been quite horrific. (1989: 112)

In 1993, Kerry Carrington, commenting on the outcomes of her research into female delinquency, wrote:

> That one in five female State wards end up in detention at some stage before turning eighteen is a dreadful indictment on a welfare system that takes children into care but has, in fact, a long history of providing very little care . . . It should not be surprising that it is unsupported youth (that is State wards, homeless youth and girls living in incestuous or intolerable family environments) who are most vulnerable to detection for petty delinquencies. (Carrington 1993: 146–47)

It would seem that little has changed for Australia's young people. A recent New South Wales Community Services Commission report demonstrated that:

> children in NSW State care through no fault of their own were at least 15 times more likely to end up in a juvenile jail than other children . . . female wards were 35 times more likely to enter a juvenile detention centre than other girls. (YSA V16, no. 1 1997)

That a significant proportion of young people taken into state care find themselves incarcerated as criminals towards the end of their childhood years, when the state begins to withdraw guardianship support, begs careful and considered analysis. Clearly current policy and practice is not working. In spite of glaring awareness of the inadequacies of the welfare system in caring for young people, the state seems to have been able to offer little by way of structural change, at the very least, for young women unable to reside with their families. It would seem that social work and welfare practitioners, such as myself, as agents advocating for the rights of these young women, have been unable to implement substantive change using established practice theories. Perhaps the time to turn to alternative theoretical frameworks for understanding and addressing social disadvantage such as homelessness is upon us. Feminist practice faces some particularly confronting challenges. As a feminist I can attest to this.

PRACTICE/THEORY DILEMMAS

Few of the young women I worked with felt that the women's movement had anything to offer them. Some suggested that, if anything, feminism made them feel less adequate because they couldn't identify with the independent, well-paid, educated, childless, politically astute, powerful image they carried of feminists. Such stereotyping of feminism undermines what feminists have been trying to achieve, and yet many of the *feminists* with whom young female service users came into contact appeared on the other side of a counter or desk—or, if not a physical divider, a psychological one. In the eyes of the young women, these service providers not only appeared to have *their* lives sorted out, but *they* were earning substantial wages, and presented—although not deliberately, and often in spite of active effort to overcome differences—as having everything the young women wanted and needed: a job, a home, money, an education and power (over the young women). Many of the young women could not even imagine themselves in such positions, much less relate to the workers as fellow human beings. One young woman in a workshop with representatives from the Department of Social Security burst out: 'We don't see you as human, you don't understand what it's like to be unemployed' (Jenny, 16 years).

How can feminist social work practice reconcile such contributions, albeit unintentional, to women's oppression? A frequently repeated complaint by the young women was that they were sick and tired of being 'pushed around and told what to do by everyone'—men and women alike, particularly professionals who controlled access to social security benefits and welfare services.

It is not surprising that feminist social work practice does not always fit comfortably with youth homelessness work. What could be more apt than for young women themselves to point this out? In the broader arena, the women's movement has been called to account for marginalising particular groups of women, such as non-English speaking, black and lesbian women (Stanley 1990), largely on the basis of its white, middle-class public face. Diversity within academic feminist writing, driven by debates over sameness and difference within feminism itself and between individuals and groups of women (Wearing 1996), has given rise to a plethora of *new* feminisms.

After initially reeling at this theoretical field resembling a tangled mass, I found the ambiguities, challenges and tensions strangely reassuring and ultimately useful. Many of the dilemmas encountered by feminist youth workers over attempts to measure gender discrimination against class- , race- and age-based disadvantage and oppression were effectively addressed in this opening up of feminist dialogue.

As a researcher and practitioner, I had to come to terms with transience, change and uncertainty as they are embodied in both lived experience and theory. There were continual challenges in reconciling my own theoretical and political agenda with the everyday material, psychological and emotional survival needs of young people who saw little relevance in feminist practice and theory at best, and treated feminism as an enemy at worst. This was particularly played out in attempting to locate and define points of nexus between the young women's needs and the feminist cause of overcoming *all* women's oppression.

I had to recognise that aspects of established feminisms such as radical, Marxist, socialist and liberal did not always translate comfortably into either my own life or youth work. It was difficult to accept the homogenising effects created by assumptions around oppression and being female, political loyalty, 'less vulnerable/more powerful' models for reconstructing femaleness, interpretations of the family as necessarily oppressive for women, and lack of acknowledgment of diversity among women. Although these characteristics of various feminisms are based on the shared experience of many women and have been politically necessary and effective, rigid adherence to any singular, prescribed or defined code for being a *feminist* or a *woman* has the same potential to abuse power as a patriarchal social order.

The young women I worked with, whilst victims of abusive experiences, were also victimisers. They perpetrated acts of violence and aggression towards males and females across all age groups. The feminist explanation that this violence resulted from personal, collective and structural victimisation was useful for explaining some aspects of their behaviour. However, this was ultimately disempowering and limited, because the defining rationale was the young women's victim status. As a worker, I suspected that these young women were not behaving violently just as a reaction to their own abuse experiences, which many of them shared—which many women and men share. It seemed that their development of a repertoire of violent behaviours could also be linked to both deliberate deviation from traditionally gendered classist roles prescribing appropriate and acceptable behaviour for young women and a construction of femininity emerging from their own cultural locations. Further to this, many of the young women wanted a family life: they aspired towards partnering, having babies and *homes*. Amongst many reasons, they wanted— as most generations do—to improve on their parents' efforts, to *get it right*. Social work theories based on psychological and sociological explanations tend to pathologise these aspirations, because contemporary culture has other *duties* for young women to perform. (Having given birth to four children myself, I wonder whether there is ever a time in a woman's life that makes motherhood and parenting a sensible thing to do.) Aspects of feminist poststructural theorising offer clues towards reaching some understanding of how these young women resisted victimisation while highlighting how feminist practice might unintentionally contribute to processes of subjugation.

PEEPING THROUGH THE KEYHOLE OF POSTSTRUCTURALISM

Michel Foucault's work on subjectivity and power challenges structuralist understandings of natural order, fixed truth, the human subject, knowledge and the operation of power. Foucault, amongst other poststructural theorists such as Derrida, Lyotard and Baudrillard, views people as subjects who variously adopt resistant or compliant behaviours, depending on where and how personal advantage, survival and control are perceived to be derived (Weedon 1987). Individual subjectivity is seen as non-fixed and shifting, changing according to situations, circumstances and expectations which are contextualised within a social, cultural and political framework of regulatory control mechanisms that exercise power in 'ideologically diffuse and institutionally disarticulate ways' (Davis 1992: 2). Power is re-read as positive and productive.

Rather than a force which finds basis at the top of a hierarchy, power is understood as operating in a 'capillary' manner through discourse, or language systems, in which knowledge, meaning and truth claims, as well as human subjectivity, are produced and perpetuated.

Foucault sees the historical development of power contributing to the production of humans as 'subjects' in three main ways (Foucault 1983: 208): first through scientific discourses which objectify humans, such as the 'criminal', the 'insane' or the 'homeless'; second through 'dividing practices', wherein 'the subject is either divided inside himself [sic] or divided from others', such as mad/insane, sick/healthy, homed/homeless; and third, through a concern with how we subjectify ourselves, such as through sexuality, the proposition being that the invention of the soul ensured self-regulation by placing governmentality within ourselves.

Poststructuralism recognises, however, that with power's 'will to produce' there are inevitably less favourable effects. Foucault states: 'My point is not that everything is bad, but everything is dangerous' (Rabinow 1984: 343)—hence the array of inequities and injustices in the social field. As power is produced in the struggle between control and resistance, there are myriad specific locations in which to examine how these inequities occur. The potential to incite reordering of power relations exists also within these sites of contestation. Hope is fuelled in recognising that change is possible because there is no fixed natural order or truth that transcends time and place: all is contingent. However, actually achieving change can be very difficult, as Chris Weedon (1987: 7) points out:

> Social relations, which are always relations of power and
> powerlessness between different subject positions, will determine
> the range of forms of subjectivity immediately open to any
> individual on the basis of gender, race, class, age and cultural
> background. Where other positions exist, but are exclusive to a
> particular class, race or gender, the excluded individual will have
> to fight for access by transforming existing power relations.

Drawing on Foucault's concept of 'dividing practices', Weedon emphasises the importance of subjective identity. Entrenched categories such as 'insane', 'criminal' or 'homeless' impose defining social, cultural and juridical codes which operate to limit and constrain subjective choices while maintaining the status quo. For example, having been defined as 'a homeless person', an individual must work against a range of powerful social and cultural discourses to rid themselves of this identity. Given that people who are homeless are marginalised by their social and economic position, they have a considerable—and not always surmountable—task in moving into a more central subjective position, such as 'employed with a mortgage'.

Foucault's (1981) third claim, that individuals are self-governed by regulatory technologies imposed on the body through the discourse of sexuality, has found alliance with feminism's concept of the 'politics of the body' (Bordo 1993: 185). Both schools of thought claim that the body has been appropriated as a site of control. The feminist movement's theoretical and practical concerns with the sexualising and objectifying of women's bodies through the male/female dualism is supported by Foucault's assertion that sexuality is a discursive construct imbued with the intent of policing and controlling human subjects. This concept of the body as a regulatory site offers some assistance in the attempt to address the chain of abuses experienced by some young women, such as sexual and physical assault, exclusion from home and family, criminality and prostitution. That these young women often turn assault on to themselves in the form of substance abuse and self-harm behaviour is no surprise if we understand their subjectivity as shaped by abuse of their physical body. Many of these young women locate personal power and control within this domain of physical and sexual violence.

FEMINIST POSTSTRUCTURAL THEORISING

[Feminist poststructuralism] becomes feminist firstly when matters of femaleness and maleness and the differences and dominations between and within them are made a central feature of analysis and secondly, when analysis implies a challenge of some sort to any inequitable relationships of power which involve gender or sexuality. (Kenway 1992: 5)

Rather than perceiving male hegemony deriving from structural top-down patriarchy, feminist poststructuralism sees the subjugation of women as a result and function of discursively constructed differences between men and women, not feminine and masculine essentialism (Weedon 1987; Sawicki 1991). A poststructural reading of gender and resistance illuminates the binary category female/male and the cultural meanings attached to and surrounding such constructs and their historical locations, while a feminist lens allows us to identify and focus on male privilege and manipulation of power. For poststructuralism to have useful application for feminists, acknowledgment of power's attachment to the gendering of meaning cannot be overlooked.

Some feminists (see Wearing 1996; Ramazanoglu 1993) have expressed concern that deconstruction of categories such as man/woman, white/black, heterosexual/lesbian, in the cause of diminishing difference as a reason for privileging one group over another, will result in de-politicising and dissipating subjective positions in which disadvantage is located and from which collective strength can be gained. In this vein, Betsy Wearing (1996) argues for a retention of the category 'Australian women' (1996: 54). As this chapter makes explicit, I also suggest that differences between and within groups must be recognised. There might not be fixed subjectivity, but there are shared moments, experiences and locations of disadvantage along a range of dividing and intersecting axes. Young women experiencing homelessness, while retaining individual subjectivity, constitute a specific historical category representing a range of social disadvantages. To discard this identification would be to risk rendering their cause invisible.

A poststructural reading of subjectivity as a multiplicity, with no necessarily fixed identity, is useful for examining the options available to these young women for recasting and redefining their social positioning. Poststructural feminists do not seek to ascribe or define a standard code for being female, but instead assert that an infinite range of options is and should be available to women. As Wearing (1996: 48) outlines: 'The socially produced body is not a fixed, immutable body, the body as "thing", it is a metaphoric body where meanings are constantly reproduced, but are also in flux.' Using these concepts, the challenging, various, self-destructive, often violent and 'anti-female' behaviours of the young women, even though to a degree forced (because survival may depend on it) and chosen (because it was an empowering option), could be read as legitimate constructions of femininity, and not deviations at all.

VICTIMISING PRACTICES

In their studies of homeless youth, both Gordon Tait (1992) and Nanette Davis (1992) call on poststructural theory. Tait urges youth workers to 'reassess' definitions of homeless youth as the subcultural group 'street kids'. He suggests that such categorisation is constructed 'at the intersection of a wide range of governmental strategies' through 'rituals of truth' that are used to legitimise the control and policing of homeless young people

(1992: 12–17), while at the same time providing a measure for identifying 'normal', 'well adjusted', 'non-deviant' youth.

Davis's (1992) application of a Foucauldian concept of social control asserts that 'homeless female youth' are subjected to further processes of gendered victimisation which operate in two main ways: 'systemically' through social institutions—in particular, juridical, educational and welfare systems—and 'directly' through interpersonal interaction (1992: 2), such as sexual assault.

Leslie Harman (1989), studying interactions between workers and residents in women's shelters in Canada, found that shelter workers reinforced and rewarded traditional gender role behaviour amongst residents. My own observation in accommodation facilities revealed that behaviour amongst young women which deviated from feminine 'norms' incited negative and marginalising responses from workers and peers (Crinall 1993). Young women's domesticity and passivity were reinforced and rewarded, while physical strength, dominance and domestic uselessness were considered endearing and useful characteristics in young men.

Fortunately, many of the young women, aware of their victimisation by and within a system that was meant to be assisting and caring for them, knew they had to confront and negotiate the world and its players in ways different from privileged homed adolescents. Their responses were ingenious, inspiring and sometimes tragic, as anyone who has worked with young people in crisis will know. In adopting challenging and defiant ways of being female, the young women demonstrated their ability to resist victimisation and practise power. Of course, some young women complied with traditional and more conservative femaleness, as a choice that worked—albeit ephemerally—for them. Moving between various subjective options is an effective strategy in retaining choice of multiple subjective positions, thereby exercising control in both resistance and power play.

CONCLUSION

In order to explore how we might address interpersonal practices that contribute to the perpetuation of narrow subjective options for young women, a poststructural approach emphasises *how* this happens, rather than *what* happens (Brennan 1995: 101). In resisting docile, right, moral and desirable *good girl* behaviour, young women experiencing homelessness become, in the words of Davis (1992) and Connell (1987), 'the ideal victim'. As 'violators of gender role norms and social expectations of the feminine', they are treated unequally due to gender, age, class, race, religion and ethnicity (Davis 1992: 1). Workers need to be cautious of participating in similar processes of victimisation. By working with individuals as *homeless victims*, rather than as active resistors and survivors, we contribute to the construction of their victim status. In our work with these young women, perhaps we might best assist by confirming and encouraging their ability to devise strategies of resistance and empowerment; to do otherwise could shade our practice with dogmatism, classism and ageism.

As feminist social welfare workers, we need to be prepared to continuously evaluate our work practices with awareness of the multifarious sites and forms abuse, oppression, victimisation and subjugation take. This may lead us to explore locations and practices not necessarily indicated by the mainstream women's movement, or identified through instituted feminist frameworks. We need to remind ourselves of Kerry Walker's (1991) caution: little is achieved for young women escaping violent and abusive situations if the form and location taken by that abuse and oppression are all that changes.

Gender justice in the field of youth homelessness requires consistent emphasis, promotion and articulation from committed individuals and groups. Incorporation into a multiplicity of perspectives is required, including work practice, policy formation and broader social supports that are able to not only wend and weave their way through the maze of resistances, but to establish new pathways. Feminism can work in partnership with a poststructural understanding of how difference, power, control and resistance work can guide us, but we need to further our understanding of how these might come together. This will happen if workers are prepared to challenge their own assumptions and expectations of the forms that resistance can take, what being female means and how the processes of victimisation seek to locate in individuals, categorising and constructing them as victims. Re-examining how power is dispersed and exercised through the truth claims of knowledge reveals that an array of social, political, economic and cultural mechanisms contribute to the construction of young women as *homeless* subjects. We must ask how we perpetuate this defining category. Whose construct is it? I doubt it is the invention of young people unable to reside with their families.

We must listen to the wisdom of young women who are homeless while sharing the advantages of our own subjective positionings, actively engaging in the reciprocity of the relationship. Practice wisdom tells us that prescribed formulae for successfully overcoming life crises are not necessarily useful, as grand theories of social work practice might have us believe.

Eroding the boundary between worker and client by rejecting such dualisms as privileging, dividing and essentially excluding constructs is perhaps the first step in declaring there is much that young women already offer feminist social welfare practice.

REFERENCES

Alder, C. and Sandor, D. (1989) *Homeless Youth as Victims of Violence,* Criminology Research Council, Canberra

Beauchamp, T.L., Faden, R.R., Wallace, R.J. and Walters, L. (eds) (1982) *Ethical Issues in Social Science Research,* John Hopkins University Press, Baltimore

Bordo, S. (1993) 'Feminism, Foucault and the Politics of the Body', in C. Ramazanoglu (ed.), *Up Against Foucault: Explorations of Some Tensions Between Foucault and Feminism,* Routledge, London

Brennan, C. (1995) 'Beyond Theory and Practice: A Postmodern Perspective', *Counselling Values,* January, vol. 39, pp. 99–107

Carrington, K. (1993) *Offending Girls: Sex Youth and Justice,* Allen & Unwin, Sydney

Community Services Victoria (1989) *Children and Young Person's Act, Vic.,* Melbourne

Connell, R.W. (1987) *Gender and Power,* Allen & Unwin, Sydney

Crinall, K. (1993) What Can Feminism Offer Young Homeless Women?, Master's thesis, Deakin University, unpublished

——(1995) 'The Search for a Feminism that Could Accommodate Homeless Young Women', *Youth Studies Australia,* vol. 14, no.3, pp. 42–47

Davis, N. (1992) 'Systemic Gender Control and Victimisation Among Homeless Female Youth', paper presented at the National Centre for Soci-Legal Studies, La Trobe University, Melbourne

Dreyfus, H. and Rabinow, P. (eds) (1983) *Michel Foucault, Beyond Structuralism and Hermeneutics,* Chicago University Press, Chicago

Foucault, M. (1978) *The History of Sexuality—Volume 1: An Introduction,* Penguin Books, London

——(1983) 'The Subject and Power', H. Dreyfus and P. Rabinow (eds), in *Michel Foucault, Beyond Structuralism and Hermeneutics,* Chicago University Press, Chicago, pp. 208–20

Gardiner, K. and O'Neil, M. (1987) 'What's A Nice Girl Like You Doing in a Place Like This?: A Report on Young Women's Access to Youth Housing', a discussion paper prepared by the National Youth Coalition for Housing (NYCH), Canberra

Gillespie, P., Roberts, M. and Watson, S. (1990) *Girl's Talk: Young Women Talk About Housing,* Zig Zag Young Women's Resource Centre, Brisbane

Gordon, L. (1986) 'Feminism and Social Control: The Case of Child Abuse and Neglect', in J. Mitchell and A. Oakley (eds), *What is Feminism?* Pantheon Books, New York

Green, S. (1993) *Our 'Voluntary' Homeless*, Children's Welfare Association of Victoria Inc., Melbourne

Harman, L.D. (1989) *When a Hostel Becomes a Home*, University of Western Ontario, Toronto

Healey, K. (1993) 'Gender and Discrimination' in K. Healy (ed.), *Issues for the Nineties*, vol. 18, Spinney Press, Sydney

Hirst, C. (1989) *Forced Exit*, Salvation Army, Melbourne

Human Rights and Equal Opportunity Commission (1989) *Our Homeless Children*, Report of the National Inquiry into Homeless Children, Australian Government Printing Service, Canberra

Kenway, J. (1992) 'Making "Hope Practical" Rather Than "Despair Convincing": Some Thoughts on the Value of Poststructuralism as a Theory of and for Feminist Change in Schools', paper delivered to the Annual Women's Studies Conference, Deakin University, Geelong

Mitchell, J. and Oakley, A. (eds) (1986) *What is Feminism?*, Pantheon Books, New York

National Youth Coalition for Housing (NYCH) (1990) *Do You Come Here Often? Another Report on Women and Supported Housing*, Canberra

Nielson, J. (ed.) (1989) *Feminist Research Methods: Exemplary Readings in the Social Sciences*, Westview Press, Boulder, Col.

Oakley, A. (1981) 'Interviewing Women: A Contradiction in Terms', in H. Roberts (ed.), *Doing Feminist Research*, Routledge, London

Rabinow, P. (ed.) (1984) *The Foucault Reader: An Introduction to Foucault's Thought*, Penguin, London

Ramazanoglu, C. (ed.) (1993) *Up Against Foucault: An Exploration of Some Tensions Between Foucault and Feminism*, Routledge, London

Roman, L. (1989) Double Exposure, unpublished paper, Education Faculty, University of Wisconsin, Maddison

Salvation Army/Crossroads (1993) Report of The Bridge Program, unpublished paper, Melbourne

Sawicki, J. (1991) *Disciplining Foucault: Feminism, Power and the Body*, Routledge, London

Stanley, L. (ed.) (1990) *Feminist Praxis*, Routledge, London

Stanley, L. and Wise, S. (1990) 'Method, Methodology and Epistemology in Feminist Research Processes', in L. Stanley (ed.), *Feminist Praxis*, Routledge, London

Tait, G. (1992) 'Reassessing Street Kids: A Critique of Subculture Theory', *Youth Studies Australia*, vol. 11, no. 2, pp. 12–17

Taylor, J. (1990) *Giving Women Voice*, Brotherhood of St Laurence, Melbourne

Tong, R. (1998) *Feminist Thought*, 2nd edn, Allen & Unwin, Sydney

Walker, K. (1991) Untitled and unpublished keynote speech delivered at 'A Strong Link in the Chain: A Conference about Young Women', Melbourne, November

Walkerdine, V. (1990) Deakin University Distance Education Study Materials, video tape

Wearing, B. (1996) *Gender: The Pain and Pleasure of Difference*, Longman, Melbourne

Weedon, C. (1987) *Feminist Practice and Post Structuralist Theory*, Basil Blackwell, Oxford

Young Women's Housing Collective (YMHC) (1991) *Do You Feel Safe Here? A Study of Young Women's Experiences in Youth Housing and Refuges*, YMHC, Melbourne

6 Offending mothers: Theorising in a feminist minefield
Lee FitzRoy

INTRODUCTION

The sexual assault of a child by her/his mother is a rare and serious indictable crime. It has been estimated that 97–98 per cent of sex offenders are men (Finkelhor 1986; ABS 1994, 1996). However, these texts do not identify the statistical occurrence of women sex offenders. Therefore, we can assume that women comprise the remaining 2–3 per cent of sex offenders.

This chapter seeks to present some of the current theoretical frameworks which I have found useful when thinking about the issue of women who have perpetrated sexual violence. These analyses include writings from feminist, postmodern and feminist psychoanalytic theorists. In exploring their contribution to the complex and difficult issue of women's use of sexual violence, I have resisted the temptation to provide over-arching explanations which may simplify what is a very dense and political subject. Instead, I hope this work will be a useful contribution to current debates on women's violence.

This form of sexual violence has largely been denied or minimalised within feminist theorisations of sexual assault (Hall and Lloyd 1988; Kelly 1988; Bass and Davis 1995). Feminist theory has understandably focused on the sexual violence perpetrated by men; however, this has led to an absence in the feminist discourse on the sexual violence perpetrated by women. I would suggest that there are a number of pertinent reasons why this form of violence should be addressed by the feminist discourse.

Initially, there is a legitimate requirement for feminist theory and the sexual assault field to actively engage with and validate the experiences of those women and girls who have experienced sexual violence perpetrated by women. As my previous research has focused on the experiences of women survivors, I feel unable to comment on the experiences of men or boys who may have been sexually assaulted by their mothers or other female caregivers (see Elliott (1993) and Saradjian (1996) for further discussion). Although the victim/survivors of female violence are few in number, their experiences have generally been defined as marginal to the experiences of victim/survivors of male violence. Through acknowledgment and research, feminist theory could name and legitimatise the experiences of 'different' victims of violence, and further explore the issues related to offending women.

The second reason is that the existence of this form of sexual violence leads us to examine more closely complex questions regarding the nature and exercise of power; the use of sexual violence; the construction of femininity and masculinity; the intersection of class, culture and gender in the experiences and choices of women; and the place of children within our families and communities.

Because of the controversy which surrounds such views—or, in other words, the 'feminist minefield' one enters when acknowledging the phenomenon of offending mothers—I would like to briefly discuss some personal and professional dilemmas which emerged during this research.

REFLECTIONS ON MY EXPERIENCE OF THE FEMINIST MINEFIELD

I have incorporated a feminist analysis into my personal life and professional work for many years and the majority of my work has been with victim/survivors of male violence. Whilst working in the sexual assault field, I met and worked with two women who disclosed their experiences of child sexual assault perpetrated by their mothers. Due to the absence of such experiences within the mainstream sexual assault literature, I sought to undertake my own research into the phenomenon.

This research led me to a number of theoretical questions concerning women's sexual offending behaviour; however, such questions were compounded by personal and professional dilemmas. To briefly summarise, I had serious personal doubts about committing time, energy and resources to a project which focused upon a very small number of women who perpetrated sexual violence. Given the horrific litany of crimes perpetrated by men against women and children, I feared that my work would be misused to futher oppress or blame women. However, amidst lingering doubts, I now return to my commitment to the rights of women and children and my feminist analysis of power. This commitment leads me to question the effects of the traditional power hierarchies upon women and their relationships with 'other' women, children and men. Consequently, I would suggest that my work can be understood as a contribution to a critical body of knowledge which seeks to name and understand other experiences of oppression.

This research has demanded that I, as a middle-class, educated, white, academic woman, acknowledge the position of power from which I speak (Spivak 1987) and the abuses of power that I have implicitly and explicitly enacted over others (Flax 1990). Whilst researching women's offending behaviour, it has been important to reflect upon my own investment in an idealised view of myself as the perfect woman, feminist worker, daughter and potential mother (Maynes and Best 1997). In addition, the process of unpacking a dominant feminist discourse on women, power and violence has also challenged my investment in 'innocent knowledge' (Flax 1990), which was the assumption that I would discover an essential 'truth' about women's use and abuse of power. I am aware that I was hoping for a truth which would exonerate women of responsibility for their actions.

My search led me to two conflicting theoretical positions which I sought to reconcile. These theoretical positions will be discussed later in the chapter. After consulting with an insightful theorist, I was encouraged to critically engage with this conceptual paradox and to further demonstrate the possible links between these two conflicting positions. In writing this chapter, I have sought not to reconcile such positions, merely to present some insights from different bodies of knowledge which I have found useful and which led me to further research. In addition, I have been challenged to question my need for a singular 'truth' which would excuse women—or indeed provide a neat and universal explanation as to *why* women would perpetrate sexual violence. In searching for this truth, I found myself seeking essentialist explanations which totalised women's experiences of patriarchy and violence and simplified how such experiences were incorporated into their sense of self and consequently their actions. Initially, I argued an essentialist reason for 'why' women would enact sexual violence against the bodies of their children. However, the reality is that, as I am in the very early stages of my research into women sex offenders, I am unable to offer any clear explanations as to why this form of violence occurs. However, I do feel that I am able to offer some contribution to the difficult issues and questions which emerge.

Along with this challenge, I have had to engage with my

fantasy of the 'perfect mother' (Chodorow and Contratto 1989), which highlighted the difference between my response to child sexual assault committed by mothers as compared with sexual violence perpetrated by fathers. In thinking about the actions of a mother/offender, I found myself locating the mother as victim, which reflected the traditional feminist view of women acting from a place of oppression.

Aside from my personal response, I need to acknowledge my awareness of the political and ideological context within which this research is located. I fear that any public discussion of women's offending behaviour may negatively affect the gains of the feminist movement. The gains to which I am referring include the social and political acknowledgment that sexual violence is a gendered crime whereby 98 per cent of perpetrators are men and that this violence against women and children emerges explicitly from a phallocentric social context. My concern about a possible backlash against women's services is also linked to my awareness of the current conservative political and economic context, where direct services for victims of violence are increasingly being mainstreamed, outsourced and privatised (Hughes 1996; Wilson 1996). I am concerned that any research which addresses women's offending behaviour may be used by a neo-conservative government to further marginalise women's services. However, I would suggest that a number of workers are currently grappling with the issue of women's violence within human service organisations. Workers in the child protection, mental health, youth housing, domestic violence, sexual assault and criminal justice systems have identified a number of difficult issues and creative strategies that emerge from their work with violent women (FitzRoy, 1997).

FEMINIST ANALYSIS

Second-wave feminism has offered us a broad body of knowledge which demonstrates the oppressive nature of the social, political, economic, historical and discursive context within which women live. Clearly, this context is one which severely curtails the power exercised by women, thus affecting their opportunities for 'real' choice, as distinct from constructed or socially defined choices. Therefore, when we use a mainstream feminist analysis, we can very clearly see the position of oppression and powerlessness within which a woman offender is located, and which may inform her choice to offend. The resulting difficulties which arise through the use of such a contextualisation process will be explored shortly.

An additional element within our understanding of the choices made by individual women is the real possibility that the majority of women sex offenders are also victim/survivors of child sexual assault, adult rape and/or domestic violence (McCarty 1986; Saradjian 1996). The theoretical and practical issues raised by this issue are very complex and I do not wish to suggest that a cycle of violence theory is an appropriate theoretical framework to assist us in making sense of women's offending behaviour. As evident in the broad body of feminist literature on child sexual assault, we know that the vast majority of women who are sexually assaulted as children do not enact sexual violence against their own children. However, it does remind us to ask more complex questions about the impact of oppression upon the oppressed and how these experiences are manifested and enacted in the lives of the victim.

This leads us to the issue of women as 'victims'. The difficulty in viewing women solely as oppressed is that we are unable to view the actions of the woman/offender as arising out of an individual choice to assault the other person. Consequently, the woman as offender—her intention, ability and choice to 'act'—as well as the crime and the victim herself are rendered invisible (Wolfers 1992). This is an extremely problematic outcome for victim/survivors, workers and feminist theory. As survivors have informed us, some mothers do make choices to enact sexual violence against their daughters and, although we can contextualise the position from which women make this choice, their choice to enact a crime still exists. As Smart (1994: 28) comments: '"choice" is, of course, an inadequate term, but it does allow for agency'. In acknowledging choice, it is important, however, to problematise the notion of 'choice' further, given the complex interplay of class, sexuality, ethnicity and gendered identity. In other words, I am reflecting upon the different understandings and experiences of power, and consequently the levels of 'choice', amongst diverse groups of women.

In seeking to make sense of women's choices, I have found the work of Featherstone (1997) and Parker (1995, 1997) very useful. In reflecting upon the child protection field, Featherstone (1997) draws upon Parker's (1995) analysis of the ambivalent relationship mothers may have with their children. Parker posits that some mothers share a love/hate relationship with their children; however, due to social taboos about mother hate, this ambivalence is hidden.

As identified previously, the dichotomised construction of woman and consequently 'mother' as either victim or offender, but never both, exists as an inherently problematic point for traditional feminism. Within a traditional analysis of gender, the view that masculinity is the primary problem has meant that mainstream feminism has been unable to critically engage with the relationships of power and domination that exist between women and their children or 'other' women. Assisting us to move forward from this point is the theoretical legacy of feminism, juxtaposed with a postmodern analysis of the construction of gendered identity. This body of knowledge tells us that women are constructed within a fundamentally patriarchal and ethnocentric historical and social context. Therefore, we can acknowledge that women, like men are socialised within a hierarchical social order, where they learn to categorise other members of society into oppositional dichotomies and enact forms of oppression against these 'others'. I am not suggesting that these forms of abuse are always overt or violent in action; merely that some women participate in, benefit from and perpetuate power relationships which maintain the dominant capitalist and patriarchal order. Therefore, as Kelly (1991: 15) comments: 'Taking social construction seriously, including the fact that women do not live outside patriarchal ideologies and practices, means we can locate women as abusers within feminist analysis—but it is complicated.' Through the use of a critical feminist and postmodern perspective, we can clearly locate women's offending behaviour within an analysis of the 'relations of domination' (Flax 1990: 182). Using this theoretical framework, such violence could be seen as a possible outcome of a social and historical context which legitimatises the abuse of those defined as inferior others and which condones the use of sexual violence as a weapon to dehumanise and degrade this other.

In acknowledging the construction of women within a phallocentric discourse, it is not a difficult step to recognise that women could abuse power in the private realm of the family. In reality, the family may be the primary place where many women can feel both a sense of power and have the opportunity to enact power against an 'other'—a child (Kelly 1991). Feminist theorists have developed a detailed body of knowledge which contextualises the enacting of physical violence and infanticide by mothers against their children (Parton 1990; Wise 1990; Featherstone 1996; Riley 1996).

However, it is important for us to problematise the different responses women offenders experience when they come into contact with the child protection and criminal justice systems. Clearly, as women of colour have argued, race and class issues may fundamentally affect how the child protection and criminal justice systems view mothers and the specific interventions into 'other' women's child-rearing practices. I think it is important for us to acknowledge that women of colour, working-class women, lesbian or disabled women are examples of other women who experience the intense scrutiny and regulation of their child-rearing practices (Walkerdine and Lucey 1989).

In relation to sexual offences, much anecdotal evidence leads me to the conclusion that women are rarely charged with sex offences within the criminal justice system. However, if a woman is charged and found guilty of sexual offences against her child, she is more likely to be pathologised as a 'monster' within the public discourse and receive a far more severe sentence compared with male sex offenders. This obviously relates to the 'madonna/ whore' (Welldon 1988) or 'victims/villains' (Featherstone 1996) dichotomy, whereby some women, once they breach the boundaries of traditional motherhood, are punished far more severely than male offenders.

Such issues remind us to critically analyse the different ways in which child rearing and child abuse are constructed and defined across cultural, class, historical and social boundaries. Therefore, it is reasonable to assume that different women may experience power and enact violence in a variety of ways, depending on their subjective experience and location with our social reality. This reflection leads me to explore some of the useful insights from postmodern theory.

POSTMODERN ANALYSIS

Postmodernism offers us a critical analysis of both the nature of power and the 'truth' of the notion that masculinity and femininity are fixed essential categories (Flax 1990; Nicholson 1990; Sawicki 1991; Butler 1993; Everingham 1994; Featherstone and Trimble 1997). These analyses offer a challenge to the traditional assumptions of what or who is a 'man' or 'woman'. Of particular interest to me is the manner in which postmodernism also challenges the essentialised notion that masculinity is homogeneously 'aggressive', which exists in oppositional terms to a 'passive' femininity. These critical questions assist us in identifying that there are specific discursive or language-based practices which construct a very particular form of gender identity. These practices also attribute the enacting of sexual violence to an essentialist view of a hegemonic or dominant masculinity (Kelly 1991; Liddle 1993; Smart 1994; Connell 1995; Featherstone and Trinder 1997). As we can see, this dominant view fails to acknowledge the possibility that women can enact sexual violence against others. Smart (1994: 28) made the following observation:

> The location of 'bad' sexuality with the homogeneous masculine has meant that women have been denied any responsibility for their own harmful behaviour. Women's (sexual) violence has perhaps been feminism's 'best kept secret' and we need to develop further the means of analysing it rather than denying it.

Therefore, postmodernism, in a similar manner to feminism, offers us a critical analysis of the political and historical construction of masculinity and femininity. Postmodernism rejects the strict binary opposites such as man/woman, public/private, subject/object. Instead, postmodernism argues that women take up contradictory positions and roles within a variety of public and private spaces. For example, a working-class woman from a Judao-Christian background may experience discrimination within the employment market; however, within her own community, she may enact a form of structural or personal racism against another working-class woman who is a practising Hindu. In this new conceptual space, we are able to see that women, as individual agents, take up diverse and changing roles within their communities and families.

Although feminism has sought to validate the differences amongst women, it has been bound by the hierarchical and binary opposites inherited from modernity. This theoretical legacy has disallowed feminism the opportunity to explore the contradictory position of a woman who may be both a victim of male oppression and who has chosen to enact oppression against an 'other'. A feminist postmodern analysis would argue that, instead of a fixed view of women as either victim or villain, women's subject positions could be viewed as fluid, contradictory and dynamic. Using this analysis, we can see that women may be located in conflicting and contradictory positions within multiple discourses (Hollway 1989). As Featherstone and Trimble (1997: 152) comment: 'This approach is deeply critical of theories of socialisation that assume that societal norms about masculinity and femininity are transmitted in a straightforward way.' Postmodernism extends our current understanding of the mechanisms of power which construct gender identity. In addition, it enables us to ask complex questions about the impact of such constructions upon the lives and choices of women. If we accept a feminist analysis of historical and social power relations, then we can also identify that women, as a result of shifting positions of power and vulnerability, may also exercise or abuse power.

POSING SOME QUESTIONS

Clearly this brief overview of some of the contributions of feminist and postmodern theory has enabled me to place useful pieces of the jigsaw on the table. I believe this theoretical contribution enables us to ask different questions about women and mothering. We are led to interrogate the different ways in which women encounter and experience gender, class and race oppression and/or interpersonal violence. In addition, it also leads us to ask a variety of different questions as to how the intersection of these multiple facets of women's subjectivity impact upon women's understanding and experience of power and their use or abuse of sexual violence.

Within this discussion, feminist psychoanalytic theory may provide some additional understandings of women's constructed and lived experience. I will briefly identify a number of intersecting issues which have emerged from this complex body of theory.

Feminist psychoanalysis has identified the issue of blurred bodily and emotional boundaries between mothers and daughters (Flax 1990; Hollway 1997; Parker 1995, 1997). I spoke to a few women who identified as survivors of child sexual assault perpetrated by their mothers. The women commented that they had no sense of where their mother's body ended and their own body began. As Phoenix commented: 'I was her property. To do what she wanted [with] and in a sense for her, her daughter must have been an extension. Because I was basically a part of her that she controlled and manipulated' (quoted in FitzRoy 1997: 46).

The blurred boundaries between mother/perpetrator and daughter/victim may result from the process of gestation, birth, breastfeeding and a shared biological and gendered identity. The intersecting issues of both the possession of the daughter as a 'part-object' of the mother (Welldon 1988) and the resulting blurry boundaries between mother and daughter lead me to consider this issue as an area for further research.

Saradjian (1996) completed a study of over 50 women sex offenders and proposes a speculative theoretical model. This model is based on the assumption that women who sexually assault children do so because they have 'learnt through experience that this behaviour can meet what they perceive to be their needs' (1996: 187). The needs listed by Saradjian include power and control, and sexual and affiliation needs (1996: 194). The issue of sexual needs which are met by sexual violence is a difficult one for feminist theory to engage with due to the traditional feminist analysis which has de-emphasised the sexual nature of male violence. This issue, along with the role of 'desire' within sexual violence perpetrated by men and women, remains unresolved in feminist theorising and would benefit from further investigation. To explore further the notion of unmet needs, I have begun to ask questions about the possible link between women enacting sexual violence against the bodies of their children and the issue of women enacting self-mutilation against their own bodies. A number of authors have explored the issue of self-mutilation (Solomon and Farrand 1996) and the possibility that women may view their child as a 'part-object' (Welldon 1988) or a 'substitute self-object' (Wolf 1988). Whereas, in men, the act is aimed at an outside part-object, in women it is usually against themselves, either against their bodies or against objects they see as their own creations: their babies (Welldon 1988: 8).

Along with questions as to how women view their bodies and the bodies of their children, we are left with the question as to why the violence is sexualised. In thinking about this issue, there are unanswered questions concerning to the impact of childhood experiences of sexual violence and how these experiences may be incorporated within a woman's understanding of self, power, agency, identity and needs. These questions remain for me and form part of my theorising on how different women may engage with, make sense of and experience oppression.

In seeking to theorise why the violence is sexualised, I find myself returning to a feminist analysis of the act of rape. To penetrate the body of the child, with objects or fingers, is an extremely invasive form of violence, whereby the one who penetrates invades the body of the 'other', thus becoming powerful within our social order. The victim may be objectified, dehumanised and annihilated (Welldon 1988; Saradjian 1996) through the actions of the perpetrator. We can question whether this process of annihilation is relevant or significant to our understanding of mother/child rape.

BRINGING FEMINIST, POSTMODERN AND PSYCHOANALYTIC IDEAS TOGETHER

Earlier, I discussed how I had fallen into a modernist trap—that is, I found myself seeking an essential truth as to why a mother would sexually assault her child. During this chapter, I have drawn on specific aspects of feminist, postmodern and psychoanalytic theory and tentatively suggested some useful conceptual links between these diverse theoretical frameworks. To summarise, feminism offers me a complex analysis of the construction of 'women': gendered power relationships and the phallocentric basis to sexual oppression. Postmodernism offers me a way of conceptualising the multiplicity of subjective realities which may affect different women's sense of self: experience of the body; understanding of familial and intergenerational experiences; and their notions of mothering, rights, power and identity. Such diverse experiences could consequently affect their level of 'choice' within their families or the social world. Psychoanalytic theory has enabled me to ask a range of questions about how different women may make sense of their world and their experiences, and how such experiences may be manifested in their lives. I would suggest that drawing together elements of these theoretical analyses provides a useful contribution to future theorising about the issue of sexual violence perpetrated by women against their children.

CONCLUSION

This chapter has sought to present some ideas and possible bodies of knowledge which may be useful when thinking about and working with mothers who have sexually assaulted their children. I have explored some specific insights which are assisting me in my current research on women sex offenders. At this stage in my research, these musings are purely speculative; however, they encourage me to think more critically about the fluidity of power relations and the diverse subject positions which women inhabit within our social world.

Given the complexity of the issues inherent within this discussion, I am hesitant to make definitive comments as to the possible implications for social work practice. However, I would suggest that different practice strategies could emerge from an expanded discursive and theoretical space. This space could allow for the often-contradictory reality of women's lives, their experience of ambivalence within mothering and their capacity for agency and/or violence to inform the direct practice of workers in a number of fields. In addition, the possible intersection of issues which emerge for workers (the majority of whom are women: daughters and/or mothers) could also be addressed and incorporated into the development of an ethical practice model. Along with the shifting of these previously fixed discursive boundaries comes a necessity for human service agencies and the child protection and criminal justice systems to address the often-contradictory responses enacted against offending mothers.

These are complex issues that would benefit from further discussion and research. I believe this chapter is a small contribution to such debates amongst workers who are concerned about the perpetration of sexual violence within our community.

REFERENCES

Australian Bureau of Statistics (ABS) (1994) 'Court proceedings initiated by police', Canberra, cat. no. 45012
——(1996) 'Women's safety survey', Canberra, cat. no. 41280.
Bass, E. and Davis, L. (1995) *The Courage to Heal: A Guide for Women Survivors of Child Sexual Abuse,* 3rd edn, Harper Collins, New York
Butler, J. (1993) *Bodies That Matter: On the Discursive Limits of 'Sex',* Routledge, New York
Chodorow, N. and Contratto, S. (1989) 'The Fantasy of the Perfect Mother', in N. Chodorow (ed.), *Feminism and Psychoanalytic Theory,* University of Yale Press, London
Connell, R. (1995) *Masculinities,* Allen & Unwin, Sydney
Elliott, M. (ed.) (1993) *Female Sexual Abuse of Children—The Ultimate Taboo,* Longman, London
Everingham, C. (1994) *Motherhood and Modernity: An Investigation into the Rational Dimension of Mothering,* Open University Press, Milton Keynes
Featherstone, B. (1996) '"Victims or Villains"? Women who Physically Abuse Their Children', in B. Fawcett, B. Featherstone, J. Hearn and C. Toft (eds), *Violence and Gender Relations: Theories and Interventions,* Sage, London
——(1997) '"I Wouldn't Do Your Job!": Women, Social Work and Child Abuse', in W. Hollway and B. Featherstone (eds), *Mothering and Ambivalence,* Routledge, London
——(1998) 'Taking Mothering Seriously—The Implications for Child Protection', unpublished paper presented at the 2nd International Conference on Social Work in Health and Mental Health, Melbourne, January
Featherstone, B. and Trimble, L. (1997) 'Domestic Violence and Child Welfare', *Child and Family Social Work,* vol. 2, pp. 147–59
Finkelhor, D. (1986) *A Source Book on Child Sexual Abuse,* Sage, Beverly Hills
FitzRoy, L. (1997) 'Mother/Daughter Rape: A Challenge for Feminism', in S. Cook and J. Bessant (eds), *Women's Encounters with Violence: Australian Experiences,* Sage, Thousand Oaks, Cal.
——(1998) Offending Women: Conversations with Workers, unpublished paper
Flax, J. (1990) *Thinking Fragments: Postmodernism, Feminism and Psychoanalysis,* University of California Press, Berkeley
Hall, L. and Lloyd, S. (1989) *Surviving Child Sexual Assault,* Falmer Press, London
Hollway, W. (1989) *Subjectivity and Method in Psychology,* Sage, London

——(1997) 'The Maternal Bed', in W. Hollway and B. Featherstone (eds), *Mothering and Ambivalence*, Routledge, London

Hughes, D. (1996) 'Coping with Contracting', *Community Quarterly*, no. 41, pp. 37–41

Kelly, L. (1988) *Surviving Sexual Violence*, Polity Press, Cambridge

——(1991) 'Unspeakable Acts', *Trouble and Strife*, vol. 1, pp. 13–20

Liddle, A.M. (1993) 'Gender, Desire and Child Sexual Abuse: Accounting for the Male Majority', *Theory, Culture & Society*, vol. 10, pp. 103–26

Maynes, P. and Best, J. (1997) 'In the Company of Woman: Experiences of Working with the Lost Mother', in W. Hollway and B. Featherstone (eds), *Mothering and Ambivalence,* Routledge, London

McCarty, L. (1986) 'Mother–Child Incest: Characteristics of the Offender', *Child Welfare*, vol. 65, no. 5, pp. 447–58

Nicholson, L. (ed.) (1990) *Feminism/Postmodernism*, Routledge, London

Parker, R. (1995) *Torn in Two: The Experience of Maternal Ambivalence*, Virago, London

——(1997) 'The Production and Purposes of Maternal Ambivalence', in W. Hollway and B. Featherstone (eds), *Mothering and Ambivalence*, Routledge, London

Parton, C. (1990,) 'Women, Gender Oppression and Child Abuse', in Violence Against Children Study Group (eds), *Taking Child Abuse Seriously*, Unwin Hyman, London

Riley, A. (1996) 'Murder and Social Work', *Australian Social Work,* vol. 49, no. 2, pp. 37–43

Saradjian, J. (1996) *Women Who Sexually Abuse Children: From Research to Clinical Practice,* John Wiley & Sons, London

Sawicki, J. (1991) *Disciplining Foucault: Feminism, Power and Body,* Routledge, London

Smart, C. (1994) 'Law, Feminism and Sexuality: From Essence to Ethics', *Canadian Journal of Law and Society*, vol. 9, no. 1, pp. 15–38

Solomon, Y. and Farrand, J. (1996) 'Young Women Who Self Injure', *Journal of Adolescence*, vol. 19, no. 2, pp. 108–21

Spivak, G.C. (1987) *In Other Worlds: Essays in Cultural Politics*, Methuen, London

Walkerdine, V. and Lucey, H. (1989) *Democracy in the Kitchen: Regulating Mothers and Socialising Daughters*, Virago, London

Welldon, E. (1988) *Mother, Madonna, Whore: The Idealisation and Denigration of Motherhood,* Free Association Books, London

Wilson, K. (1996) 'Demysifying the Tendering Process', *Community Quarterly,* no. 41, pp. 42–43

Wise, S. (1990) 'Becoming a Feminist Social Worker', in L. Stanley (ed.), *Feminist Praxis: Research, Theory and Epistemology in Feminist Sociology,* Routledge, London

Wolf, E. (1988) *Treating the Self: Elements of Clinical Self Psychology,* Guilford Press, London

Wolfers, O. (1992) 'Same Abuse, Different Parent', *Social Work Today*, vol. 23, no. 26, pp. 16–22

7 Deconstructing masculinity—reconstructing men

Bob Pease

The purpose of this chapter is to examine the implications of the current debates about the relationship between postmodernism, critical theory and feminism for emancipatory practice with men. I will outline the implications of the postmodern challenge to feminism by deconstructing 'men' and will demonstrate how a recognition of variations among men is central for understanding men's lives and for reconstructing men's subjectivities and practices. I will also argue that the critical postmodern notion of the discursive production of multiple subjectivities has considerable potential for providing guidance to men about how their subjectivities and practices have been constituted and how they can be transformed.

POSTMODERN FEMINISM AND THE CRITICAL STUDY OF MEN

In recent years, feminist theories have all been interrogated by feminist postmodern and poststructural perspectives. There has been considerable debate about the implications of these interrogations for the feminist project of the emancipation of women (Weedon 1987; Spelman 1988; Nicholson 1990; Scott 1988; Hirschman 1992). Little attention, however, has been given to the implication of these debates for the critical investigation of men. In this chapter, I will explore the implications of postmodern feminism for theorising and changing men.

While being mindful of the dangers identified in the feminist debates about essentialism and difference in relation to the category of 'women' (Fuss 1987; Soper 1990; Evans 1990), I am interested in what we can learn from these debates about the category 'men'. If we question the constituency of 'women', I would argue that we must equally question the constituency of 'men'. If there is progressive potential in unpacking the term 'women', why not unpack 'men' too? The 'men' of white feminism have too often been white, middle-class men, for women who wanted equality with men did not seek equality with non-white men (Phelan 1991: 128). Thus we should avoid lumping all men together in a uniform category and, when discussing men, we should remember *which* men we are talking about.

To deconstruct 'men' as a category enables us to identify that the supposedly fixed position between anatomical sexuality and gender stereotypes can be broken. We may be more able to legitimate behaviours that do not seem to derive from one's sex. Thus the progressive potential of a postmodern perspective would be to reveal alternative modes for the construction of masculinities not yet realised (Saco 1992: 39). Ironically, some feminists suggest that the progressive possibilities for deconstruction may be greater for men than for women. Weedon (1987) argues that it is important for men to deconstruct masculinity and the role that it plays in the reproduction of patriarchal power. She claims that this is politically more important for men—who have claimed an objective rationality—than it is for women, whose voices have been marginalised by this discourse (1987: 173).

Kristeva (1981) argues that only men can put in jeopardy their symbolic position, because only they are subjects with a position to subvert. As men have had their 'Enlightenment', they can more easily afford a sense of decentred self and a humbleness regarding the truth of their claims, but for women to adopt such a position would weaken further what has never been strong (De Stefano 1990: 75). Indeed, one cannot deconstruct something that has never been fully granted, whereas men have not been denied the status of subject (Braidotti 1987: 237). Thus I would argue, along with Best and Kellner (1991: 208), that 'certain strands of postmodern theory can be used to deconstruct ideologies of male domination'.

DECONSTRUCTING MEN AND MASCULINITY

How to theorise men has been a major source of disagreement among women, with much of the early feminist critique resting on a categorical model of gender that regards men as a monolithic identity.

How meaningful is it to talk about men as an homogeneous category? How relevant is it to refer to men as a collectivity with a unitary set of interests? What are the implications of a categorical approach to men? For example, talking about men's interests suggests that all men can be taken as a group in which most or all men are essentially the same. So when it is said that it is in men's interests to maintain gender inequality, does this refer to *all* men or only a specific group of men? When it is said that men control the mode of reproduction, are *all* men being referred to? What about gay or anti-sexist men? When it is said that men dominate the public sphere, are all men or a particular circle of powerful men with exclusive interests being identified (Brittan 1989: 108, 198)?

Are all men violent and are all men potential rapists? Answering this affirmatively can produce a sense of guilt, despair and paralysing self-hatred in men (Seidler 1991: 131). It leaves little room for men to change. Men are even able to accept this view of themselves as a justification for doing nothing, since it appears to be a facet of their nature.

One of the difficulties with the sentence 'Men oppress women' is that it makes oppression definitional of men. It implies that men oppress women by virtue of being men. If, instead, we say things like 'Men oppress women because they control the institutions of the state', or 'because they exploit their labour in the home', or 'because they use power and control tactics with them', it seems to imply a possibility for change. If we define men solely as oppressors, all that men can do is to will their own demise as men (Middleton 1989: 9, 13).

Furthermore, can we assume that all behaviour that takes place between men and women is determined by that one, general gender-based group relation (Middleton 1992: 150)? To talk about gender relations between men and women distracts our attention from issues such as race and class. We should always keep in focus *which* men and *which* women we are talking about.

DIVERSITY AND DIFFERENCE IN MEN'S LIVES

We are now entering a new stage in which variations among men are seen as central to the understanding of men's lives. Thus we cannot speak of masculinity as a singular term, but rather should explore masculinities. Men are as socially diverse as women and this diversity entails differences between men in relation to class, ethnicity, age, sexuality, bodily facility, religion, world views, parental/marital status, occupation and propensity for violence (Collinson 1992: 35).

Differences are also found across cultures and through historical time. Connell (1992: 3) has pointed out that the discourse about 'masculinity' is constructed out of 5 per cent of the world's population of men, in one region of the world, at one moment in history. We know from ethnographic work in different cultures how non-Western masculinities can be very different from the Western norm.

Most of the literature on men and masculinity focuses on middle-class professionals and managers and the lives of these men are often taken as representative of masculinity *per se*. But power is not shared equally among men and men's class locations influence the nature of their dominance over women.

In addition to the class bias in the men and masculinity literature, there is also a presumption of whiteness in discussions of men's lives. To address this imbalance, we have seen in recent years, in North America and the United Kingdom, accounts of masculinity written from the perspective of black men and men of colour (Staples 1989; Gordon 1993; Mercia and Julien 1988).

Furthermore, very few books written by heterosexual men have seriously attempted to come to grips with gay liberation arguments. Moreover, most do not acknowledge that mainstream masculinity is heterosexual masculinity. From the gay viewpoint, heterosexual masculinity is a privileged masculinity that is created and maintained by homophobia at the expense of homosexual men and women (Nierenberg 1987: 132).

Research suggests that men undergo changes throughout the life cycle in relation to their experience of their bodies and in relation to aggression and dominance, as well as shifts in value orientations (Thompson 1994). These changes have implications for how men position themselves in relation to women.

Men also differ markedly in terms of how they position themselves in relation to feminism. Connell notes from the men he has interviewed that responses range from 'essentialist rejection' to 'wary endorsement' to 'full blown acceptance' (1991:15). Clearly men vary in their level of awareness of their oppressive role in relation to women. Organised responses range from men's rights groups which deny that men have power in society and men's liberation groups where women's issues disappear completely as men search for the 'deep masculine', to profeminist responses, where men embrace the feminist analysis and publicly support women's struggles (Kimmel 1987: 272–80).

MEN AND GENDER POWER

The implications of the preceding analysis demonstrate the extent to which the study of masculinities is a study of power relations. Many of these different masculinities stand in different relations to power. Hearn (1989: 90) describes this in terms of 'hierarchic heterosexuality', to acknowledge that some men are more power-ful than others. Connell (1987: 92) distinguishes between hegemonic masculinity and various subordinate masculinities. Some men are in positions where they can impose their particular definitions of masculinity on others in order to legitimate and reproduce the social relations that generate their dominance.

Thus, although large numbers of men benefit from patriarchy, they do not all benefit equally. Middle-class, white, heterosexual masculinity is used as the marker against which other masculinities are measured (Kimmel 1997: 61). When Hearn (1992) set out to investigate the ways in which men maintained and reproduced their power in the public sphere, he made it clear that he was referring especially to able-bodied, heterosexual, middle-aged, middle/upper-class, white men (1992: 3). Such men not only dominate women, but also dominate different types of men—for example, heterosexual men dominate gay men; upper-class men dominate working-class men; white men dominate men of colour. This domination does not necessarily involve a conscious process of exploitation (although, of course, it may); it exists because of the relative privileges to which heterosexual, upper-class, white men have access.

Clearly, forms of bonding *across* class, race and ethnic lines operate at the expense of women (Kimmel 1987: 61). Men in general are advantaged through the subordination of women, although, ethnographically speaking, different men are advantaged in different ways. This does not, however, deny the existence of 'anomalies' consistent with the global subordination of women. There are sites where women hold power over men or are at least their equals. The intersection of gender with class, sexuality and race relations produces sites where dominant–subordinate rela-tions are more complex—for example, where white heterosexual women are employers of working-class men, patrons of homosex-ual men or politically dominant over men of colour (Carrigan et al. 1987: 90). Thus, while not all men have power in relation to all women, all men are embedded in power relations.

IMPLICATIONS OF DIVERSITY AND DIFFERENCE FOR THEORISING MEN'S POWER

Because white, middle-class, heterosexual men have had no clearly identifiable common enemy to organise against, they have had little incentive to explore diversity and differences (Orkin 1993: 22–23). Furthermore, as the more powerful group, these men have no power-maintenance reasons to explore differences amongst themselves. White, middle-class, heterosexual men are the ones who have created various 'others' on to whom their own repressed parts can be projected. This group of men has most difficulty in acknowledging its multiplicity and so identifying with others (Hollway 1989:130).

Pratt (1984), in her autobiographical narrative of a woman who identifies as a white, middle-class, Christian-raised, Southern lesbian, explores how her white identity was based on the marginalisation of differences within and without. Lorde (1984: 115) describes how we have been socialised to respond to difference in one of three ways. At first we ignore it if we can; if that is not possible, we tend to copy it if we think it is dominant, or destroy it if it is subordinate. It is not the real differences between us that separate us, but rather our own refusal to recognise the differences and to avoid the distortions that arise from misnaming them (1984: 115).

There is a connection between marginalised and oppressed people and 'marginalised and oppressed parts of ourselves' (Ingamells 1994: 3). The more people acknowledge multiple parts of themselves, the more they will be able to identify with different positions (Hollway 1989: 129). So, when men come to appreciate difference between and within us, we are likely to be more open to the shifts involved in attending to, for example, feminist and anti-racist claims. The categories of 'men' and 'white' and all that they represent are thus more likely to be challenged (Ferguson 1993: 179–80).

Where else does this acknowledgment of diversity and difference in men's lives lead us? It could be said that there are problems when we extend a deconstructive analysis from feminism to the politics of masculinity (Middleton 1989: 14). When criticised by women, men have been very quick to say that one cannot generalise and that all men are different. A common defence among men has been that if all of what women say about men is not true for *them*, then none of it is true. This extreme inductivism is the opposite danger to essentialist deductivism.

The question is whether the recognition of differences between men means that we lose sight of men as a gender? Some would argue that it is not relevant to consider differences in men's experiences, as we may distract attention from *all* men's culpability in the oppression of women (Orkin 1993: 23). Segal (1990: 205) points out that recognising a plurality of masculinities does not in itself address the social and political domination of men over women. I am aware of the danger of 'pluralised masculinities becoming a new and perhaps more sophisticated means of forgetting women' (Collinson and Hearn 1994: 8).

I would argue, however, that to critique the notion of a homogeneous category of men is not to deny the reality of systematic gender inequality. The fact that men are divided among themselves along ethnic and class lines, and enact competing versions of masculinity within the same class or ethnic group, only makes the task of analysis more difficult (Brittan 1989: 141). Indeed, 'the power and domination of men over women persist in many diverse ways, partly through these differences' (Hearn and Collinson 1994: 115).

Thus emphasis on diversity and difference 'ought not to degenerate into a diversified pluralism that gives insufficient attention to structured patterns of gendered power, control and inequality' (Collinson and Hearn 1994: 10). Differences among men can only be understood with reference to the structure of the gender order and the recognition of multiple masculinities does not reduce the sociology of masculinity to a postmodern kaleidoscope of lifestyles (Connell 1992: 736). Clearly, we must avoid the danger of losing sight of patriarchy.

One way to avoid this danger is to theorise men simultaneously 'along two axes, the male–female axis of men's power over women within the marginalised groups, and the male–male axis of non-hegemonic men's relative lack of power *vis-a-vis* hegemonic men' (Brod 1994: 89). This is consistent with Collinson and Hearn's (1994: 11) exhortation that 'both the unities and differences between men and masculinities as well as their interrelations' should be examined.

THE DISCURSIVE PRODUCTION OF MASCULINITIES

Men's experience of class, race, sexuality, age and ideology constitutes their social identity. This social identity can be understood as being formed through competing discourses. Discourses make positions available for individuals and these positions are taken up in relation to other people. When taken up, the world is seen from the standpoint of that position and this process involves, among other things, positioning oneself in relation to categories and story lines. It also involves locating oneself as a member of various sub-classes of categories as distinct from others. So one develops a sense of oneself 'as belonging to the world in certain ways and thus seeing the world from the perspective of one so positioned' (Davies and Harre 1990: 46–47). Through this process, people can become *fixed* in a position as they are shaped by 'the range of linguistic practices available to them to make sense' of the world (Potter and Wetherall 1987: 109).

The individual is thus constituted and reconstituted through a variety of discursive practices and changing material circumstances. The relevance of this notion for emancipatory practice with men is that men can reconstitute themselves through a self-conscious and critically reflective practice.

It is within discourses that we are offered subject positions, which convey notions of what it is to be a man or a woman and which constitute our masculinity and femininity (Weedon 1987: 100). Thus masculinity is not an inherent property of individuals. Rather, we learn the discursive practices of society and work out how to position ourselves as 'male' of a certain type (Davies 1989: 13). Our masculine sense of ourselves is historically provided in a series of social practices within different discursive frameworks. Within these frameworks, we are invited to take up or turn down different subject positions and a sense of masculine identity that goes with them. That is, each framework enables men to think of themselves as men in particular ways (Jackson 1990: 268).

There is no single patriarchal discourse of masculinity, and a number of contradictory ones are currently available to men. On the other hand, discourses are not all equal in relation to what men '*as subjects* may have invested in them; some subject positions are more compelling for men than others' (Saco 1992: 24). In this context, hegemonic masculinity may be considered as a dominant discourse.

As discourses compete with each other for the allegiance of individual subjects, however, the accommodation of subjects to particular discourses is never final and is open to challenge and change. Thus the nature of masculinity is one of the key sites of discursive struggle for men (Weedon 1987: 97–98). As people *choose* positions in discourses, I am interested in the question as to why men choose to position themselves as patriarchal subjects in the gender discourses in which they participate. Why is it that some men take certain positions in a discourse rather than another? Under what conditions will men choose to position themselves as non-patriarchal subjects in their discourses? What accounts for the difference between men?

One answer to these questions is that it is a combination of emotional investment and vested interests in the relative power the position offers (Saco 1992: 35). Hollway (1984: 237) acknowledges that it is in part a result of investments and returns resulting from such discourses, but she also argues that it is a result of the available positions offered by discourses. The relevant implication is that increasing the range of subject positions in a discourse will open up more opportunities for change in men's lives.

Thus, to sum up, masculine subjectivity is understood as a

process involving constant negotiation of multiple subjectivities, or fragments thereof, in which men have unequal investments—for example, a man's social identity may comprise being a white, upper-class, heterosexual man. Some identities will be prioritised over others, as 'in a divided society it is very difficult to hold on to numerous composite identities equally at the same time' (Hearn and Collinson 1994: 111).

Postmodernism, then, decentres the self and promotes the notion of multiple selves (Jackson 1990: 40). Multiple subject positions resulting from involvement in different discourses lead to individual men being composed of a set of contradictory positionings or subjectivities. This multiplicity of discourses leads to internal conflict and contradiction.

AGENCY AND THE FORMATION OF NEW SUBJECTIVITIES FOR MEN

An essential premise of this chapter is that it is necessary to avoid discourse determinism, whereby individuals are mechanically positioned in discourses, leaving no room to explicate the possibilities for resistance and change (Henriques et al. 1984: 204). While subjectivity is constructed within discourse, subject positions cannot be predicted as the outcome of specific discourses. Dominant discourses can be resisted and challenged, and this resistance is an important stage in the development of alternative subject positions.

Thus we need to develop ways of encouraging resistance. The possibility of agency is opened up to the subject by 'the very act of making visible the discursive threads through which their experience of themselves as specific beings is woven' (Davies 1993: 12). Some resources must be available, though, for the individual to have agency. These include: a definition of oneself as one who makes sense of the meanings within discourses; access to alternative discursive practices; access to means of bringing about alternative positionings; a belief in one's capacity to reposition oneself and access to others who will support alternative positionings (Davies 1990: 359–60).

While individuals may, under certain circumstances, resist their particular positioning in dominant discourses, these opportunities are shaped by the availability of alternative discourses. One needs, then, to have knowledge of more than one discourse and to recognise that meaning is plural. This enables some degree of choice on the part of the individual, but 'in order to have a social effect, a discourse must at least be in circulation' (Weedon 1987: 106, 110).

In this view, one brings about social change through 'the production of new discourses and so new forms of power and new forms of self' (Ramazanoglu 1993: 24). Even if the possibility of generating new discourses does not exist, and a choice of alternative discourses is not available, it is still possible to resist dominant discourses (Weedon 1987: 106). One is able to do this by working on the contradictions between old and new discourses.

Thus resistances are expressions of contradictions resulting from the exercise of power. Feminism is regarded as a counter-discourse that resists 'the hegemony of male domination [and] utilises the contradictions in these hegemonic discourses in order to effect their transformation' (Hekman 1990: 190).

It is my point that the contradictions in patriarchal discourses provide the starting point *for men,* as well as women, to generate counter discourses. Men's subjectivity is equally contradictory and while men may have a lot to lose by responding to feminism, they also have much to gain, because of the limitations imposed by hegemonic masculinity on their own lives. Furthermore, as women change their positions in patriarchal discourses, the repercussions will interrupt men's positioning as well (Hollway 1982: 502–503).

I am arguing in this chapter that the postmodern concept of the decentred subject has greater critical potential for provoking inner change in men than the humanist notion of an innate self. The aim is to decentre the dominating self of traditional masculinity and allow the possibility of fragmented and contradictory multiple selves (Jackson 1990: 268–69). Thus the task is to destabilise and denaturalise 'the scripts in place and create the space for a variety of different masculinities to be performed' (Gutterman 1994: 234). The progressive potential of this analysis would be to reveal alternative possibilities for the construction of masculinities not yet realised (Saco 1992: 39). Profeminism is one such masculinity that has yet to be fully realised.

MEN, FEMINISM AND EMANCIPATORY PRACTICE

Many women have questioned the genuineness of some men's apparent support for feminism. They have argued that there is frequently a large gulf between commitment to egalitarianism in principle and in practice (Thomas 1990: 153). Feminists can only judge men's words and actions, but some feminists regard all male praise of feminism as a takeover bid in disguise (Moi 1989: 184).

Given that men have for centuries denied women the opportunity to have their own space and time to build solidarity, they cannot expect that, all of a sudden, women will appreciate some men's willingness to examine their own experience (Tolman et al. 1986: 66). Following Burghardt (1982), who confronted this dilemma as a white man working to end racism, I believe that the resolution of this conflict resides in praxis (1982: 111). As a man, I can be involved in fighting sexism and still be viewed as sexist by women, which is an understandable perception for women to have about men. The dilemma can be resolved as profeminist men's activities reveal that they are not as sexist as some women thought and as, through their anti-sexist practice, they discover elements of sexism still with them that need attention.

Of course, because of our dominant subject position within patriarchy, forming an alliance with feminism(s) will never be a simple matter. Men's practices in acting against patriarchy will always be problematic, as we do not occupy the same position in relation to the dominant power structures as women (Hearn 1992: 15, 230). On the other hand, there are men who have endeavoured to live according to egalitarian and non-sexist principles. Such men stand in contrast to other men, who have not made the slightest concession to feminism (Brittan 1989: 182). I would argue that these men do not have the same interests as other men, nor do they share the same identity. There is more to us than categories. We have an integrity that cannot be captured in those terms (Phelan 1991: 133). While men cannot *not* be oppressors, we can do things differently (Hearn 1987: 167). It is thus important to analyse men in terms of their individual and collective practices.

Many of men's positive responses to feminism have been personal and private matters. Men have been able to develop a less oppressive sexuality, become more nurturing in their relationships, abandon violence, take responsibility for child care and housework and confront power and control issues in their personal relationships (Hearn 1989: 168). They are able to make significant changes when they begin to recognise the limitations and potential destructiveness of traditional masculinity (Pasick et al. 1990: 170). Men can change to make their lives more satisfying and live longer when they learn how their gender socialisation contributes to stress, relationship difficulties and health problems (Allen and Gordon 1990: 132).

Of course, men are also criticised for over-emphasising this area of change. Most of the current literature about men has a psychological focus. The orientation is on therapy and the use of the healing metaphor to address issues such as the father 'wound' and crises of emotions and personal meaning. Men's anti-sexist politics have been overshadowed by the more personalised and depoliticised concern with men's emotions and men's roles. The focus on men's problems in their relationships with women and other men and with themselves potentially deflects responsibility from their oppressive behaviours, and consequently men can find a way to do nothing (Stoltenberg 1991: 8–9).

The structural dimension and strategy, however, should not ignore altogether that there will be emotional consequences for men which need to be addressed. Where men's self-esteem is built on a disproportionate access to resources, establishing relations of equality will of necessity initially result in feelings of loss of self-esteem, which is something men will need to come to terms with.

Only a few heterosexual men have moved beyond personal change processes to search for a collective politics of gender among men and have recognised that they need to speak out against men's violence against women. Promoting collective responsibility among men to end men's violence is a central principle of many profeminist men's public practice. Profeminist men have been involved in the prevention of rape, speaking out against pornography, working to end battering, opposing the military and organising in support of women's reproductive freedom.

In Australia, Men Against Sexual Assault (MASA) has been involved in the organisation of forums on issues like pornography, militarism, sexual harassment and rape, conducting workshops in schools on anti-sexist masculinity for boys, producing newsletters, running workshops and giving public talks educating men about the impact of patriarchy on women's lives, speaking out in the public media about the objectification of women, and organising marches and the White Ribbon Campaign against men's violence (Pease 1997). These attempts to develop a counter-sexist politics of heterosexual masculinity have been largely confined to middle-class men and there is much to be done to relate profeminism to the experiences of working-class men. Nevertheless, profeminism for men is one of the major forms of resistance to dominant masculinity.

CONCLUSION

The most significant implication of the application of critical, postmodern ideas to the study of men is that it enables us to think critically about change in men's subjectivities and practices. It enables us to break from considering men as an homogeneous category and it helps us to understand the multiplicity of ways in which particular men dominate particular women in specific contexts. Establishing a theoretical basis for discerning these different masculinities and their different implications for the oppression of women allows for a more realistic base for the political strategy of re-forming men. Furthermore, by conceiving of these masculinities as discursive phenomena which compete with other discourses for the allegiance of individual men, there is greater potential for provoking inner change in men than the humanist notion of masculinity as an essence. The multiplicity of discourses lead to internal conflicts and contradictions for men opening up the possibilities for change.

Postmodern feminism also provides us with a way of understanding those men who do depart from patriarchal subject positions. Self-identifying profeminist men are one such group of men. A profeminist commitment among men represents a major form of resistance to dominant masculinity. Profeminist practices by men challenge the standards of identity that give men status in patriarchal discourse and allow identification of alternative subject positions for men to take up. Profeminist, straight, white men are one group of men who are rejecting hegemonic masculinity and whose lives and experiences may contribute to our understanding of the process of forming non-patriarchal subjectivities and practices. This provides an important basis upon which we can construct models of emancipatory social work practice with men.

REFERENCES

Allen, J. and Gordon, S. (1990) 'Creating a Framework for Change', in R. Meth and R. Pasick (eds), *Men in Therapy*, The Guilford Press, New York

Best, S. and Kellner, D. (1991) *Postmodern Theory: Critical Interrogations*, Macmillan, London

Braidotti, R. (1987) 'Envy or With My Brains and Your Looks', in A. Jardine and P. Smith (eds), *Men in Feminism*, Methuen, New York

Brittan, A. (1989) *Masculinity and Power*, Basil Blackwell, Oxford

Brod, H. (1994) 'Some Thoughts on Some Histories of Some Masculinities: Jews and Other Others', in H. Brod and M. Kaufman (eds), *Theorising Masculinities*, Sage, Thousand Oaks, Cal.

Burghardt, S. (1982) *The Other Side of Organising*, Schenkman, New York

Carrigan, T., Connell, R.W. and Lee, J. (1987) 'Hard and Heavy: Towards a New Sociology of Masculinity', in M. Kaufman (ed.), *Beyond Patriarchy*, Oxford University Press, Toronto

Christian, H. (1994) *The Making of Anti-sexist Men*, Routledge, London

Collinson, D. (1992) *Managing The Shopfloor: Subjectivity, Masculinity and Workplace Culture,* de Gruyter, Berlin

Collinson, D. and Hearn, J. (1994) 'Naming Men as Men: Implications for Work, Organisation and Management', *Gender, Work and Organisation,* vol. 1, no. 1, pp. 2–22

Connell, R.W. (1987) *Gender and Power: Society, the Person and Sexual Politics,* Polity Press, Cambridge

——(1991) The Big Picture—A Little Sketch: Changing Western Masculinities in the Perspective of Recent World History, paper presented at the Research on Masculinity and Men in Gender Relations Conference, Sydney, 7–8 June

——(1992) 'A Very Straight Gay: Masculinity, Homosexual Experience and the Dynamics of Gender', *American Sociological Review,* vol. 57 (December), pp. 735–51

Davies, B. (1989) *Frogs and Snails and Feminist Tales,* Allen & Unwin, Sydney

——(1990) 'Agency as a Form of Discursive Practice: A Classroom Scene Observed', *British Journal of Sociology of Education,* vol. 11, no. 3, pp. 341–61

——(1993) *Shards of Glass,* Allen & Unwin, Sydney

Davies, B. and Harre, R. (1990) 'Positioning: The Discursive Production of Selves', *Journal for the Theory of Social Behaviour,* vol. 20, no. 1, pp. 43–63

De Stefano, C. (1990) 'Dilemmas of Difference: Modernity and Postmodernism' in L. Nicholson (ed.) *Feminism/Postmodernism,* Routledge, New York

Evans, M. (1990) 'The Problem of Gender For Women's Studies', *Women's Studies International Forum,* vol. 13, no. 5, pp. 457–62

Ferguson, K. (1993) *The Man Question: Visions of Subjectivity in Feminist Theory,* University of California Press, Berkeley

Fuss, D. (1987) *Essentially Speaking: Feminism, Nature and Difference,* Routledge, New York

Gordon, M. (1993) 'Why is This Men's Movement So White?', *Changing Men,* issue 26 (Summer/Fall), pp. 15–17

Gutterman, D. (1994) 'Postmodernism and the Interrogation of Masculinity', in H. Brod and M. Kaufman (eds), *Theorising Masculinities,* Sage, Thousand Oaks, Cal.

Hearn, J. (1987) *The Gender of Oppression: Men, Masculinity and the Critique of Marxism,* Wheatsheaf, Sussex

——(1992) *Men in the Public Eye,* Routledge, London

Hearn, J. and Collinson, D. (1994) 'Theorising Unities and Differences Between Men and Between Masculinities', in H. Brod and M. Kaufman (eds), *Theorising Masculinities,* Sage, Thousand Oaks, Cal.

Hekman, S. (1990) *Gender and Knowledge: Elements of a Postmodern Feminism,* Polity Press, Cambridge

Henriques, J., Holloway, W., Urwin, C., Venn, C. and Walkerdine, V. (1984) 'Constructing the Subject', in J. Henriques, W. Hollway, C. Urwin, C.

Venn and V. Walkerdine (eds), *Changing the Subject: Psychology, Social Regulation and Subjectivity,* Methuen, London

Hirschmann, N. (1992) *Rethinking Obligation: A Feminist Method for Political Theory,* Cornell University Press, Ithaca

Hollway, W. (1984) 'Women's Power in Heterosexual Sex', *Women's Studies International Forum,* vol. 7, no. 1, pp. 63–68

——(1989) *Subjectivity and Method in Psychology: Gender, Meaning and Science,* Sage, London

Ingamells, A. (1994) Practice and the Postmodern, paper presented at the Australian Association of Social Work Education Conference, Perth

Jackson, D. (1990) *Unmasking Masculinity: A Critical Biography,* Unwin Hyman, London

Kimmel. M. (1987) 'Men's Response to Feminism at the Turn of the Century', *Gender and Society,* vol. 3, no. 3 (September), pp. 261–83

Kristeva, J. (1981) 'Women's Time', *Signs,* vol. 7, no. 1

Lorde, A. (1984) *Sister Outsider,* The Crossing Press, New York

Mercia, K. and Julien, I. (1988) 'Race, Sexual Politics and Black Masculinity: A Dossier', in R. Chapman and J. Rutherford (eds), *Male Order: Unwrapping Masculinity,* Lawrence and Wishart, London

Middleton, P. (1989) 'Socialism, Feminism and Men', *Radical Philosophy,* no. 53, pp. 8–19

——(1992) *The Inward Gaze: Masculinity and Subjectivity in Modern Culture,* Routledge, London

Moi, T. (1989) 'Men Against Patriarchy', in L. Kauffman (ed.) *Gender and Theory: Dialogues on Feminist Criticism,* Basil Blackwell, Oxford

Nicholson, L. (ed.) (1990) *Feminism/Postmodernism,* Routledge, New York

Nierenberg, J. (1987) 'Misogyny: Gay and Straight', in F. Abbott (ed.), *New Men, New Minds,* Crossing Press, Freedom

Orkin, G. (1993) 'What About the Workers?', *XY: Men, Sex, Politics,* vol. 3, no. 3 (Spring), pp. 22–24

Pasick, R. (1992) *Awakening from the Deep Sleep,* Harper, San Francisco

Pease, B. (1997) *Men and Sexual Politics: Towards a Profeminist Practice,* Dulwich Centre Publications, Adelaide

Phelan, S. (1991) 'Specificity: Beyond Equality and Difference', *Differences,* vol. 3, no. 1 (Spring), pp. 63–84

Pratt, M. (1984) 'Identity, Skin, Blood, Heart', in B. Bulkin, M. Pratt and B. Smith (eds), *Yours in Struggle: Three Feminist Perspectives on Anti-Semitism and Anti-Racism,* Long Haul Press, New York

Ramazanoglu, C. (1993) 'Introduction', in C. Ramazanoglu (ed.), *Up Against Foucault,* Routledge, London

Saco, D. (1992) 'Masculinity as Signs: Poststructural, Feminist Approaches to the Study of Gender', in S. Craig (ed.), *Men, Masculinity and the Media,* Sage, Newbury Park

Scott, J. (1988) 'Deconstructing Equality Versus Difference, or The Use of Poststructuralist Theory for Feminism', *Feminist Studies,* vol. 14, no. 1 (Spring), pp. 33–50

Segal, L. (1990) *Slow Motion: Changing Masculinities, Changing Men*, Virago, London

Seidler, V. (1991) *Recreating Sexual Politics: Men, Feminism and Politics*, Routledge, London

Soper, K. (1990) 'Feminism, Humanism and Postmodernism', *Radical Philosophy*, no. 55 (Summer), pp. 11–17

Spelman, E. (1988) *Inessential Woman: Problems of Exclusion in Feminist Thought*, Women's Press, London

Staples, R. (1989) 'Masculinity and Race: The Dual Dilemma of Black Men', in M. Kimmel and M. Messner (eds), *Men's Lives*, Macmillan, New York

Stoltenberg, J. (1991) 'A Coupla Things I've Been Meaning to Say About Really Confronting Male Power', *Changing Men*, no. 22 (Winter/Spring), pp. 8–10

Thomas, A. (1990) 'Masculinity, Identification and Political Culture', in J. Hearn and D. Morgan (eds), *Men, Masculinities and Social Theory*, Unwin Hyman, London

Thompson, E. (1994) 'Older Men as Invisible Men in Contemporary Society', in E. Thompson (ed.), *Older Men's Lives*, Sage, London

Tolman, R., Mowry, D., Jones, L. and Brekke, J. (1986) 'Developing a Profeminist Commitment Among Men in Social Work', in N. Van Den Bergh and L. Cooper (eds), *Feminist Visions for Social Work*, National Association of Social Workers, New York

Weedon, C. (1987) *Feminist Practice and Poststructuralist Theory*, Basil Blackwell, Oxford

PART III

Rethinking critical practice

8   Power and activist social work
Karen Healy

INTRODUCTION

Power, identity and change are core concepts of activist social
work. Critical social theories, such as Marxism, feminism and
anti-racist theories, provide the foundations through which these
core concepts are defined. The critical foundations of activist
social work make visible certain dimensions of social work, such
as the links between care and social control. However, it will be
argued in this chapter that these representations also suppress the
contextual and unstable character of power, identity and change
processes. In this examination, I will use critical poststructural
theory to interrogate and destabilise the critical foundations of
activist social work. Drawing on practice research from an actual
context of activist social work (see also Healy and Walsh 1997),
I will demonstrate some of the possibilities critical poststructuralism provides for depicting complexities and dynamism within
activist practice.

ACTIVIST SOCIAL WORK

I use the term 'activist social work' to refer to a diverse range of
social work approaches oriented toward radical social transformation (Fine 1992; Healy and Mulholland in press; Healy and Peile
1995; Leonard 1994). Since the late 1960s, a wide range of activist
practice models have emerged; despite their diversity, they share
theoretical foundations within the critical social science tradition.
These activist models include Marxist social work, radical
social work, structural social work, anti-racist social work, some
modes of feminist social work and radical community work, and

participatory action research. Although critical social theory is a broad terrain encompassing both modern and postmodern ideas, the critical social science school on which much activist theory is based is thoroughly modernist (Fay 1987). The modernist foundations of critical social science are evident, for instance, in the reliance of critical social work theories on notions of the 'social totality' (as seen in the heated arguments about the impact of capitalism and patriarchy on practice relations) and fixed identity (apparent in the identity politics that activists often promote). Critical social science ideas provide the terrain through which much critical practice theory is constituted and these ideas make certain strategies of analysis and action possible whilst refusing others. One purpose of this analysis, then, is to excavate and examine the critical social science assumptions which often remain unarticulated and unquestioned in activist practice theory.

CRITICAL POSTSTRUCTURALISM

Following discussion of the taken-for-granted assumptions of critical practice theory, I will consider the alternate possibilities critical poststructural theories provide for representing activist social work practice. Debate about the potential contribution of poststructuralism to critical social work theory has been slow to emerge. Indeed, many progressive social welfare theorists and policy analysts are alarmed at the apparent nihilism and potentially conservatising effects of poststructuralism (see Dixon, 1993; Taylor-Gooby 1993). Activists such as MacDonald (1996: 51) lament the growing influence of postmodernism on social theory. In her view: 'It provides the perfect rationalisation not to fight. It absolves you.' Recently, however, some thinkers within the critical social work tradition have begun to embrace—albeit cautiously—aspects of poststructuralism. In particular, Foucault's work has been used to extend the analysis of how surveillance and discipline is exercised through the human services (see Leonard 1994). By contrast, in this analysis, I use critical poststructural theory to examine and rethink depictions of critical social work practice (see also Fook, 1996; Healy and Mulholland in press; Healy and Peile 1995; Sands and Nuccio 1992).

Poststructural theories are diverse and the potential contribution of some variants of postmodernism to critical social work is, at best, limited. Indeed, Agger (1991: 9) splits postmodernism into 'apologetic and critical versions'. This analysis draws on the critical poststructural theories of Foucault and the French feminist thinkers, particularly Cixous and Kristeva. These thinkers are relevant because of their interest in activist politics and their concern with processes of power, identity and change. Foucault's work on the politics of identity formation poses a particular challenge to activist social work (see Foucault 1982, 1992). For, in contrast to activist processes aimed at forging collective identities, Foucault (1982: 785) contends that transformation involves not that we discover 'what we are' but, rather that we 'refuse what we are'. From a Foucauldian perspective, the reliance on fixed identities—even oppositional identities—reinforces the very identifications activism should aim to dismantle. Unlike critical approaches which promote the embrace of marginalised and devalued identities, poststructuralism destabilises fixed identifications. This disruptive work is intended to acknowledge the contextual variability and endless fragmentation of identity.

French feminists, particularly Cixous and Kristeva, extend and complicate poststructural approaches to identity. Although there is considerable disagreement between these two authors, both emphasise the intolerance of Western discourses to difference. In varying ways, their work demands an interrogation of activist discourses, especially the extent to which these discourses privilege rationality, mastery and unity and, in so doing, suppress non-rationality, bodily ways of knowing and sexual and racial differences (see Cixous 1994; Kristeva 1980, 1991). Both are suspicious of the reliance of modern socio-political theories on oppositional identity categories, such as 'man' and 'woman', 'middle class' and 'working class', 'white' and 'black', because these representations demand the suppression of the difference and instability that is inherent to each category. Rather than seeking to develop new and more complex categorisations, post-structuralists question the utility of identity categories altogether. For instance, Kristeva (1980: 137) emphasises the impossibility of representation as she writes: 'In "woman", I see something that cannot be represented, something that cannot be said.'

Even though Cixous and Kristeva highlight the oppressive effects of identity categories, the term 'woman' remains important to them because this category (like other disprivileged categories of Western thought) has been associated with that which Western discourses have devalued, such as the body, the irrational and the uncertain. By returning these discarded elements—that is, 'the feminine'—to language, it becomes possible to recognise difference, uncertainty, even confusion as elements of identity formation. In this chapter, I will draw on the work of Cixous and Kristeva to consider the possibilities they provide for rethinking the representations of 'workers' and 'service-users' in activist practice theories.

INTERROGATING REPRESENTATIONS OF PRACTICE

This analysis is concerned with the representations of practice in activist social theories. In particular, I will examine the representations of worker and service user identities and the implications of these depictions for apprehending processes of power and change. My purpose is to illuminate how critical social science ideas enable and constrain activist social work and to consider the possibilities that critical poststructural theory allows for representing the instability, dynamism and diversity of change-oriented practice. However, it is not suggested that either critical social science or critical poststructual theory can provide the 'truth' about what social work 'is'; indeed, such answers must be searched for in the contexts of social work practice and policy-making. Rather, my concern in this paper is to illuminate the possibilities critical poststructuralism provides for destabilising the foundational assumptions of activist theory and for opening critical social work to new possibilities for depicting activist practice.

It could be argued that the focus on the representations of activist practice theories has little relevance to the radical personal and social transformation with which activists are concerned. Yet the poststructural recognition that discourses have 'real' or 'material' effects demands of activists that they critically reflect on how we define who we are and what we do. From a poststructural perspective, discourses do not simply construct ideas, but the 'field of objects' through which the social world is experienced (Foucault 1977: 199). As Fairclough (1992: 3–4) asserts:

> Discourses do not just reflect or represent social entities and relations, they construct or 'constitute' them; different discourses constitute key entities (be they 'mental illness', 'citizenship', or 'literacy') in different ways, and position people in different ways as social subjects (e.g. as doctors and patients) . . .

From a poststructural perspective, discourses constitute what can be done, said and even thought within a given context (McHoul and Grace 1993). In other words, discourses make certain kinds of identities, social relationships and social practices possible while excluding others. Discourses are not innocent: they are fully implicated in the production of those entities they describe; hence, discourses must be recognised as a site of analysis and struggle (Fairclough 1992; Weedon 1987).

By highlighting the critical foundations of activist social work, and by refusing these ideas about the status of truth, critical poststructural theory invites new questions about practice. Critical poststructural theory can be used to contest the self-proclaimed liberatory status of activist social work theories and to consider not only what activist representations of practice make possible, but also what these depictions exclude.

CRITICAL SOCIAL SCIENCE AND THE
REPRESENTATION OF IDENTITY

A claim on which this analysis rests is that activist social work is reliant on the critical social science tradition. According to Fay (1987: 4), critical social science incorporates a range of social theories that are oriented towards liberatory social change. This broad range of social change theories includes some forms of feminism, anti-racist and multicultural theories, Marxism and liberation theology. Critical social scientists emphasise the conflictual character of society. For them, society comprises opposing forces which exist in constant struggle with each other. A key tenet of critical social science is that overarching social structures, such as capitalism or patriarchy, fundamentally order social relations at institutional and personal levels. These broader social structures determine local identities, power relations and interests. Thus, for instance, critical social science theories suggest that the relations between men and women, white and indigenous or ethnic people, able-bodied and disabled people can be apprehended only in relation to overarching structures.

The critical foundations of activist social work are evident in the assumptions about identity and power that are embraced. First, much activist theory refers to identity as fixed and determined by overarching social structures. Identities are associated with certain experiences and interests which are 'essentialist' in that 'they are said to be the necessary objective effects of pre-given social structure' (Carrington 1993: xiv). Thus, for example, groups of individuals such as women, indigenous people and people with disabilities can be said to share certain experiences by virtue of their shared social location. Furthermore, identities are classified by reference to various social categories, such as class, gender, race and ethnicity, disability and sexuality. A fundamental aim of activist social work practice is to raise awareness amongst disadvantaged people of the shared identifications and interests that are an effect of their common position(s) within broad social structures.

Second, it is recognised that individuals possess a number of identifications across a range of social categories, particularly those of class, race and gender. It is assumed that these identities overlay one another and 'add up' in the same direction (Yeatman

1993). Hence the degree of oppression experienced by an individual can be calculated according to the number of oppressed identities which they can claim. For example, Dominelli and McLeod (1989: 65) discuss the 'quadruple oppression' of race, gender, class and sexual orientation which affects black, lesbian, working-class women.

The foundational assumptions of activist social work produce specific analytic and action strategies. Activist social workers highlight the political nature of social work, which, in their view, remains concealed in orthodox practice theories. Activist practice theories are premised on the idea that welfare professionals and services users are locked in hierarchical and exploitative relationships which reflect broader social inequities. As Lowenstein (quoted in McNay 1992: 55) asserts:

> The relationship between men and women, between races, between different social classes, and between helping professions and their clients are all variations of unequal power relations in society.

The power associated with the worker's professional identity is immutable in that it is conferred through their privileged position in the social structure and their access to legitimated forms of power and knowledge. Futhermore, while workers may experience specific forms of oppression, such as those associated with gender, race, (dis)ability or sexuality, this does not erase the dominatory status conferred by their professional identity.

Activist social workers seek to enact 'a shift in power from established political, economic and cultural elites towards oppressed and powerless people' (Galper 1980: 61). Activist practice theory can be used to sensitise practitioners to the myriad of ways in which those positioned as powerless have been silenced and the extent to which workers, by virtue of their privilege, reproduce the oppression of service users. In activist practice, the authoritarian character of traditional professional relationships is replaced with a more egalitarian stance. Activist workers refuse positions of authority and seek instead to share power, knowledge and skills throughout the practice process.

Activist theory emphasises the differences between workers and users of services that can be challenged but not eradicated altogether. A fundamental contradiction of activist practice is that, regardless of the transformative strategies employed, the very presence of professional workers is disabling for service users. Ultimately, then, the most empowering thing a worker can do is to retreat from the oppressed group. Middleman and Goldberg (1974: 43) consider that a genuinely activist social worker will seek to 'work [themselves] out of a job'.

In summary, the critical foundations of activist social work pivot on the notion that there are mutually reinforcing relationships between overarching social structures, power and identity. Identity is fixed and determined by one's position within overarching social structures, and thus the 'self' is stable from context to context. Social categories such as those of gender, race and class determine one's identifications, interests and access to power. Workers and service users are depicted as opposites who, despite the identifications they may share, are locked in a relationship that is hierarchical, unilateral and oppressive. Thus, while activist workers seek to create more egalitarian practice relations, their capacity to do so is dependent on the transformation of the broader social structures under which we all live.

RETHINKING ACTIVISM: CRITICAL POSTSTRUCTURAL POSSIBILITIES

What, then, are the possibilities of poststructuralism for rethinking the representations of activist social work? In this section, I will explore this question in relation to the issue of identity in activist social work. I will begin with an outline of critical poststructural approaches to identity, followed by a consideration of its relevance to the representations of 'worker' and 'service user' identities in activist practice theories.

Many poststructuralists use the term 'subjectivity', rather than 'identity', to refer to 'the conscious and unconscious thoughts of the individual, her sense of herself and her ways of understanding her relation to the world' (Weedon 1987: 2). Poststructuralists reject the view that individuals have a fixed identity, such as that of 'woman' or 'proletariat'. Instead, subjectivity is the product of discourse and one's 'identity' varies according to the discourses operating within specific contexts. As Davies (1991: 42) asserts:

> We can only ever speak ourselves or be spoken into existence within the terms of the available discourses . . . [thus] our patterns of desire that we took to be fundamental indicators of our essential selves (such as the desire for freedom or autonomy or for moral rightness) signify little more than the discourses, and the subject positions made available within them, to which we may have access.

According to this view, subjectivities do not represent fundamental essences, but are the products of discourses. Thus, rather than privileging one aspect of subjectivity and labelling this as 'identity', it becomes possible to recognise that one may have many subjectivities—including, for example, worker, woman, mother, victim and survivor. In addition, these subjectivities are differently expressed and evaluated within specific contexts. Thus it is even possible that an identity which confers disadvantage in one context will be privileged in another (Yeatman 1995). From a poststructural perspective, then, processes of power, identity and change are represented as contextually specific, complex and unstable.

In contrast to a critical approach which seeks to encourage individuals and groups to 'reclaim the identity that the dominant culture has taught them to despise' (Young 1990: 166), poststructuralism demands attention to how discourses constitute identity. Feminist poststructuralists identify and seek to dismantle the oppositional identities on which activist politics have relied (Butler 1995; Cixous 1981, 1994; Davies 1991; Scott 1994). They are concerned that an acceptance of oppositional categories leads emancipatory theories to reproduce the very oppressions they are intended to overcome. For example, rather than support an opposition between 'men' and 'women' and embracing the latter, the work of poststructural feminists aims to dismantle this opposition. As a political tool, the destabilising process is not aimed at displacing one set of identities with a different set, but rather at creating spaces through which fluid, unstable and uncertain aspects of identity can emerge (Pringle 1995).

The notion of discourse is central to poststructural theory, and hence attention is drawn to the representation of worker and client identities in activist practice discourses. Frequently, worker and service user identities are constituted via dualistic categories such as:

- middle class/working class;
- privileged/poor;
- technical knowledge/lived experience;
- voice/silence;
- researcher/researched;
- worker/service user;
- powerful/powerless.

In activist theory, social workers are situated on the left-hand side of the dualism and service users on the right-hand side. Whilst activists seek to transcend these dualisms, the dichotomies remain central to analysis and action. As Dixon (1993: 26) contends: 'at base, we need to hold on to a major duality: the powerful and the powerless'.

The oppositional construction of worker and client identities in activist practice theories provides some important insights for practice which should not be jettisoned simply because the dualisms themselves are suspect. The dualisms demand sensitivity to the power differences between workers and service users, particularly those that arise from statutory or professional power bases. The dualisms also encourage workers to adopt a stance of humility in relation to service users and to recognise the different knowledge and experiences that they can offer for transformation. Nonetheless, poststructuralism alerts activists to the very serious simplifications on which these oppositions rely. As Fine (1994: 80) warns: 'If poststructuralism has taught us anything, it is to beware the frozen identities . . . to suspect the binary, to worry the clear distinction'.

In considering the relevance of critical poststructuralism to emancipatory practice, I will refer to practice research from an activist project in which I was involved over a two-year period (see also Healy and Walsh 1997). In this project, a core group of teenage mothers participated in researching and responding to young women's experiences of violence. Over the two years in which I collaborated on the project, I regularly collected audiotapes from the project meetings and fieldnotes about participants' and workers' reflections on the activist process in which we were engaged. In this discussion, I will analyse the possibilities of critical poststructural theory for representing different dimensions of the practice process than those which are possible to acknowledge within activist practice theory.

REPRESENTING DIFFERENCE

First, poststructuralism draws attention to the ways in which the oppositional categories central to activist practice demand the suppression of differences. For example, feminist thinkers working within the postmodern terrain have expressed concern about the extent to which the category 'woman', which is central to modern feminist theory, denies differences amongst women (Cixous 1994; Kristeva 1986). Poststructural theory challenges the constant representation of social workers and clients as opposites on the grounds that these representations occlude the complex subjectivities and histories that exist within each category.

In the activist social work project in which I was involved, it was apparent that the collective identity forged amongst the young women gave them a powerful base from which to challenge the violence they had experienced individually and collectively. Nonetheless, the group identity also created silences amongst the young women. Although there were important differences between them in their experiences of violence and its effects on them, these differences were rarely raised in project meetings. The following comments were made in a discussion with one of the young women about her experience of the project:

> *Worker:*   Did you find that other people had the same experiences as you? Did you feel less alone as a result of talking to other people—has that changed at all?
>
> *Phillipa:*   Oh sort of, but still umm, it was like totally different to everybody else.
>
> *Worker:*   Yes, yes.
>
> *Phillipa:*   Like they had, they didn't really have all the childhood stuff, not that I heard anyway.

Many of the young women in the project group had been subject to domestic violence and it was these experiences that prevailed in the group reflections on abuse. In Phillipa's view, there was little opportunity for her to discuss her experiences of violence which differed substantially from the forms of violence that dominated group discussions. Thus, although the forging of collective identifications did allow a shared base from which to speak, the forging of a collective voice demanded the marginalisation of individual voices.

Just as the collective identification of the young women as 'survivors of violence' demanded suppression of differences amongst the young women, the activist caricature of the 'powerful worker' also requires suppression of the differences amongst workers. The frequent portrayal of social workers as self-assured, arrogant and accustomed to believing that they 'can determine the best interests of others' (Ryburn 1991: 11; see also Andrews 1992; Moreau 1979) ignores the complexities and instabilities within the category of 'worker'. Feminist poststructural theory challenges the unity of the 'worker' identity by drawing attention to the impact of the body on identification (see Grosz 1994). For them, the body is a signifier enabling certain kinds of actions and prohibiting others. For instance, in contrast to the activist depiction of the powerful social work expert, there is considerable evidence to suggest that women—even within high-status professions—are often more vulnerable than their male counterparts to challenges to their professional authority (West 1995).

The importance of sexual differences in the enactment of power was acknowledged by the young women who participated in the project. These differences were highlighted during the reflection and planning sessions held once every three months, in which a mediator assisted the workers and the young women to discuss current issues and future directions of the project. Many of the young women were very aware of the different way they related to the mediator, who was male, compared with their approaches to my co-worker and I. This difference was all the more notable because of the considerable consciousness-raising around gender issues that had occurred through the project. Although the greater authority conferred on the mediator could be attributed to his role and the infrequency of his meetings with the group, one young woman reflected that his masculine subjectivity also enabled the mediator to enact specific kinds of power. As the participant stated:

> When Tony came in, everyone was totally different. Whereas sometimes we would just talk over you . . . it was like he had a whole new power that we just didn't know. It was like 'God! It's a man!' It's funny, like we bag men, but then when he came in, we respected him.

These comments highlight the fact that differences amongst workers, including sexual differences, are not incidental to the kinds of power they can exercise. At the same time, however, poststructural theory recognises that the operations of power and identity are unstable from context to context; hence it is not suggested that there is a necessary equation between specific identities and power. Rather than assuming that all differences can be reduced to a dichotomy between 'worker' and 'client', critical poststructuralism draws attention to the specific operations of power and identity within particular contexts.

REPRESENTING COMMONALITY

A second way critical poststructural theory destabilises these oppositions is by pointing to the similarities that exist between categories. For instance, in the activist literature, the oppositional identifications of workers and clients are frequently sustained through the representation of social workers as entirely naive to the lived experience of service users. As Wilson (1977: 80) asserts: 'It is hard for some social workers to imaginatively grasp the extent of hardship faced by their clients'. What this representation ignores is the importance of connection and similarity as a base for practice. Indeed, even though my co-worker and I differed from the young women participants in that, for example, neither of us had been teenage parents, we saw ourselves as personally connected to the struggles confronting the young women. Our sense of commonality with the young women, particularly our own experiences of marginalisation and violation, although different from that of the participants, provided an important motivation to work alongside the young women for change.

Similarly, the young women did not always see my co-worker and I as separate from them. The intensity of the project and the fact my co-worker and I were known to the participants prior to the project meant that subjectivities other than worker and client were recognised within the group and were fully implicated in the processes of inclusion and exclusion. For instance, my co-worker's identity as a mother was an important source of esteem and inclusion for her within the group. This esteem was often implicit in that, for example, my co-worker was included in discussions about parenting experiences. On occasion, the importance of her identity as a mother was made explicit, such as in the following excerpt taken from a discussion with a project participant.

> Robyn, was good, umm, she just I dunno, I think you've got to feel like, it was just easier with Robyn. It was just like she had kids and everything.

In this excerpt, it seems whatever differences my co-worker's status as a professional worker conferred on her, her parenting status was an important source of similarity and connection with the young women. Although I am not a parent, there were other points of commonality with the young women, such as my youth (I was only a few years older than some of the participants) and shared experiences and interests. Ironically, my professional identity was not always experienced as a threat but as a source of interest and possibly identification with the young women. Notably, since the project has been completed, a number of the participants have returned to school and one is currently studying to be a social worker!

To point to these similarities is not to gloss over the considerable differences that may exist between workers and service users. However, I am suggesting that the dualistic constitution of identity in activist practice theories suppresses points of similarity and connection which can be integral to practice processes. The representation of the powerful worker constrains the articulation of moments of shared commonality and vulnerability between worker and client insofar as it is assumed that the middle-class and professional status of the former confers a certain invulnerability upon them regardless of their experiences within the practice context and beyond it.

IDENTITY, CHANGE AND RESENTMENT

Critical poststructural theory draws attention to the disempowering effects of the oppositional constitution of worker and client identities. Although activist theory is intended to enable the oppressed to challenge the dire circumstances they face, the oppositional constitution of identity in activist practice theories leaves little room for positive political dialogue or change activity between the 'powerful' and the 'powerless'. Indeed, the danger is that, rather than enable a politics of change, the oppositional categories of activist social work foster a politics of resentment (Brown 1995; Yeatman 1993). In the politics of resentment, power is equated with domination and, as such, is seen as evil (Tapper 1993; Yeatman 1997). Power denotes a privileged structural location and the powerful are charged with being concerned only with the perpetuation of their power.

The oppositional constitution of worker and client identities in activist practice theory can promote a politics of *ressentiment* insofar as it focuses on the eradication of power rather than the analysis or transformation of how power is exercised. The critical analysis of power that was adopted within the project group supported a politics of *ressentiment*. Discussion about the diverse operations of power in the lives of the young women was effectively closed as an oppositional view of power gained prominence amongst the participants. The following reflections were recorded in my fieldnotes following a discussion with my co-worker about six months after the project began:

> Robyn [my co-worker] said it concerned her that community workers were being lumped in with police . . . Robyn felt that the accusations made by one of the young women that workers are 100 per cent bad needed to be challenged.

The equation of power with domination did not allow for a differentiation between the verbal, physical and sexual violence, such as the police violence to which some of the young women had been subjected, and the inadequate or inappropriate use of statutory power, which was the young women's main complaint about social workers. In addition, the emphasis on the eradication of all power did not enable the participants to recognise the differences between those relations of power that were firmly entrenched and those that were open to change. An oppositional constitution of worker and service user identities ignored differences between those community workers and police personnel who had demonstrated a willingness to listen to and learn from the experiences of the young women and those who willingly perpetrated abuse against them. The silences around the multiple operations of power deprived the group of strategies for dealing with the 'powerful' or for engaging collaboratively with those who have access to professional and statutory forms of power and who were willing to exercise it in favour of the young women.

The politics of resentment can also contribute to the ongoing disempowerment of service users by neglecting the forms of power to which those depicted as powerless have access. In effect, the oppositional constitution of the 'powerful worker' and the 'powerless client' effectively precludes reflection on the use of power by service users. As Yeatman (1997: 137) observes:

> When a movement understands itself as representing those who are powerless, the victims of the powerful, it neither permits itself responsibility for, nor engagement with, the affairs of the world. It maintains an innocence of worldly affairs, and, in particular, an innocence in regard to power. It does not confront the truths that power inheres in all relationships, that any interpretation of reality is in itself a manifestation of power, and that those who are relatively powerless still participate in power.

This is not to suggest that service users experience the same possibilities for the exercise of power as workers, only that activists must be alert to the possibilities that those positioned as 'powerless' in activist theory can—and indeed do—exercise power. To deny the service users' potential to use power is to denude activist theory of the complexity of operations of power within practice. For instance, feminist social workers have observed the inability of many feminist theories to acknowledge violence by women (see Featherstone and Fawcett 1994; FitzRoy 1997 and in this book). A dualistic view also denies the potential for service users to exercise power for their own empowerment. As Crinnall (1995: 45) reflects on her work with homeless young women: 'If young women are to emerge with self-worth and dignity, paradigms which argue their case on the basis of victimisation are problematic'.

Activist practice involves a tension between recognising the extent to which participants have been disempowered without confining them to the status of the 'powerless'. In the activist project in which I was involved, part of our role as facilitators was to encourage participants to recognise their capacity to exercise power. While sometimes the focus of change was on large structural and social changes, we also emphasised the participants' capacity to exercise power in the everyday activities of the project. This process involved the ongoing negotiation of power arrangements, and as such was both dialogic and, at times, highly conflictual (Healy and Walsh 1997).

One illustration of the negotiations around the operations of power occurred during a meeting at the end of the first year of the project. In reflecting on future directions for the group, one of the participants raised a criticism that she had felt excluded from the organisation of the childcare. She claimed that the workers had excluded her (and other participants) from the organisation of the childcare arrangements by failing to consult the group about hiring childcare workers and by failing to introduce the workers to the participants. Initially, my response to this criticism was one of disappointment in myself. Even though concerns about the childcare arrangements had not been raised previously, I saw myself and my co-worker as guilty of the charge the young woman made. Yes, we had organised the childcare and, yes, we had failed to introduce the childcare workers to the participants. In terms of the opposition between the powerful and the powerless, the fact that my co-worker and I had exercised power led logically to the conclusion that we had contributed to the disempowerment of the women.

Notably, my co-worker's response was different. While she affirmed the participants' questioning of the childcare arrangements and encouraged the group to consider the role they wanted to play in organising childcare, my co-worker also pointed to the young women's capacity to address some of the issues raised. The following interaction occurred in response to the young woman's criticism that the workers had not introduced the childcare workers:

> *Worker:* That's an expectation, I mean, could you go and introduce yourself and ask who . . .
> *Young woman:* But they're paid to be the people.
> *Worker:* But even when I go, when I pay for my childcare, *nobody* introduces anyone.
> *Young woman:* But the childcare was chosen.
> *Worker:* I go up to them and say, 'What's your name? My name is so and so, I'm gonna leave my child here.' I have to, every time.
> *Young woman:* But that's at a centre. I'm talking about people that are coming here.
> *Worker:* Na, anywhere.

From a critical perpective, the above interaction could appear disempowering in that my co-worker did not unquestioningly affirm the participants' voices or acquiesce to their demands, nor did she accept a view that evidence of her exercise of power corresponded to the participants' powerlessness. Rather, her response focused on how participants could address individually and collectively the concerns raised by the young woman. By refusing to place the worker centre stage in effecting change, her response pointed to some dangers of activist practice theory. There is a risk that the 'powerful/powerless' dualism of activist theory can exaggerate the power of the worker, thus making them vulnerable to blame for the failure to realise activist ideals. It can also insulate activist social work theory from critique as the failure to reach critical visions of practice relations leads not to reflection on the critical models themselves, but to reproach of workers for falling short of these ideals. By moving beyond the oppositional categories on which activist social work has relied, poststructural theory draws attention to the ongoing achievement of activist practice relations. From a critical poststructural perspective, it is not a matter of overcoming domination once and for all, but rather the ongoing negotiation of power and identity in the practice context.

If it is, as Foucault (1982: 791) suggests, that a 'society without power relations can only be an abstraction', activist practice theory must grapple with the ongoing transformation of power arrangements within the practice context and beyond it. Critical poststructural theory points to the limits of the oppositional identity categories to support the ongoing negotiation of power. By representing power as something possessed or held by one group over another, activist practice theory can suppress articulation of multiple operations of power and, most importantly, possibilities for the transformation of power relations.

CAUTIOUS CONCLUSIONS

In this chapter, I have argued that the critical foundations of activist theory suppress some of the complexities of practice and I have demonstrated some possibilities poststructuralism provides for overcoming the elisions of activist practice theories. However, I do not suggest that critical poststructuralism can completely replace the critical social science foundations of activist social work. Although limited, the identity categories of critical social science, particularly those of gender, race, class, disability and sexuality, continue to represent virulent social divisions (Walby 1992). Without these identity categories as frames of reference, the poststructural emphasis on difference and fragmentation can obscure 'the historical tenacity and material longevity of oppressive orders and structures' (Ang 1995: 67). French feminist theorists alert activists to the political dangers, but also the utility of identity (see Cixous 1994; Kristeva 1980, 1986; see also Butler 1995). Thus, even if critical workers cannot afford to jettison identity categories altogether, the work of critical poststructuralists can encourage activists to recognise the provisionality and, ultimately, the elusive character of identity.

A further concern I share with other activist social workers is the potential for poststructuralism to detract attention from structural oppression. In appraising the change potential of postmodernism, Leonard (1995) implores activist social workers not to overlook the oppressive effects of global social and economic changes on the poor and marginalised. In this chapter, I have demonstrated the silencing effects of the critical social science foundations of activist practice. The promise of 'praxis', the linking of theory and practice, which has been an attraction of critical social science, has not been fulfilled. Perhaps the problem lies not in the critical ideals in themselves, but in their often-unspoken and unquestionable position within critical social work practice theory. The 'truth' status of these critical assumptions has contributed to a monologue in which theory is privileged over practice and structural over local analyses. Often critical social work theory has been impervious to the complexities that exist within activist practice and to many of the 'conventional' practice settings where the vast majority of human service workers practise.

Critical poststructural theory can be used to prise open the critical social work canon, to demand our awareness of the foundational assumptions on which critical practice theory is based and to sensitise activists to the contradictory effects of these tenets. We need not abandon the critical social science assumptions altogether, as important political work is made possible by these ideas. Nonetheless, activists cannot afford to ignore the extent to which the representations of activist practice theories have devalued and dismissed the complexities of change in local contexts of social work practice. Critical poststructural theory supports workers to articulate the complex and contradictory interchange between the structural and local whilst resisting seeing one merely as an effect of the other. The contribution that critical poststructural theory can make at this point in the history of critical social work is to renew activist appreciation of local 'everyday' contexts of social work practice as *different*, not *inferior*, sites for building critical theories about practice.

REFERENCES

Agger, B. (1991) 'Critical Theory, Poststructuralism, Postmodernism: Their Sociological Relevance', *Annual Review Sociology*, vol. 17, pp. 105–31
Andrews, D. (1992) 'Beyond the Professionalisation of Community Work', *Social Alternatives*, vol. 11, no. 3, pp. 35–38

Ang, I. (1995) 'I'm a Feminist But . . . "Other" Women and Postnational Feminism', in B. Caine and R. Pringle (eds), *Transitions: New Australian Feminisms*, Allen & Unwin, Sydney, pp. 57–73

Brown, W. (1995) *States of Injury: Power and Freedom in Late Modernity*, Princeton University Press, Princeton

Butler, J. (1995) 'Contingent Foundations: Feminism and the Question of 'Postmodernism', in S. Benhabib, J. Butler, D. Cornell and N. Fraser (eds), *Feminist Contentions: A Philosophical Exchange*, Routledge, New York

Carrington, K. (1993) *Offending Girls: Sex, Youth and Justice*, Allen & Unwin, Sydney

Cixous, H. (1981), 'Sorties', in E. Marks and I. de Courtivron (eds), *New French Feminisms: An Anthology*, The Harvester Press, Sussex, pp. 90–98

——(1994) 'Three Steps on the Ladder of Writing', S. Sellers (ed.), *The Helene Cixous Reader*, Routledge, London

Crinnall, K. (1995) 'The Search for a Feminism that Could Accommodate Homeless Young Women', *Youth Studies Australia*, vol. 14, no. 3, pp. 42–47

Davies, B. (1991) 'The Concept of Agency: A Feminist Poststructuralist Analysis', *Social Analysis*, no. 30, pp. 42–53

Dixon, J. (1993) 'Feminist Community Work's Ambivalence with Politics', *Australian Social Work*, vol. 46, no. 1, pp. 22–27

Dominelli, L. and McLeod, E. (1989) *Feminist Social Work*, Macmillan, London

Fairclough, N. (1992) *Discourse and Social Change*, Polity Press, Cambridge

Fay, B. (1987) *Critical Social Science: Liberation and its Limits*, Cornell University Press, Ithaca, NY

Featherstone, B. and Fawcett, B. (1994) 'Feminism and Child Abuse: Opening Up Some Possibilities', *Critical Social Policy*, vol. 14, no. 3, pp. 51–80

FitzRoy, L. (1997) 'The Too Hard Basket is Full: Working with Abusive Mothers', *Proceedings of the 25th National Conference of the Australian Association of Social Workers*, Canberra

Fine, M. (1992) 'Passion, Power and Politics: Feminist Research Possibilities', in M. Fine (ed.), *Disruptive Voices: The Possibilities of Feminist Research*, University of Michigan Press, Ann Arbor, pp. 205–31

——(1994), 'Working the Hyphens: Reinventing Self and Other in Qualitative Research', in N. Denzin and Y. Lincoln (eds), *Handbook of Qualitative Research*, Sage, Thousand Oaks, Cal., pp. 70–82

Fook, J. (1996) 'Making Connections: Reflective Practices and Formal Theories', in J. Fook (ed.), *The Reflective Researcher: Social Workers' Theories of Practice Research*, Allen & Unwin, Sydney, pp. 189–202

Foucault, M. (1977) 'History of Systems of Thought', in D. Bouchard (ed.), *Language, Counter-Memory, Practice: Selected Essays and Interviews*, Basil Blackwell, Oxford, pp. 199–204

——(1982) 'The Subject and Power', *Critical Inquiry*, no. 8, Summer, pp. 777–95.

——(1992) *The Use of Pleasure: The History of Sexuality* (volume 2), Penguin, London

Galper, J. (1980) *Social Work Practice: A Radical Approach*, Prentice Hall, Englewood Cliffs, NJ

Grosz, E. (1994) *Volatile Bodies: Towards a Corporeal Feminism*, Allen & Unwin, Sydney

Healy, K. (in press) 'Participation and Child Protection: The Importance of Context', *British Journal of Social Work*

Healy, K. and Mulholland, J. (in press) 'Discourse Analysis and Activist Social Work: Investigating Practice Processes', *Journal of Sociology and Social Welfare*

Healy, K. and Peile, C. (1995) 'From Silence to Activism: Approaching Research and Practice with Young Mothers', *Affilia*, vol. 10, pp. 280–98

Healy, K. and Walsh, K. (1997) 'Making Participatory Processes Visible: Practice Issues in the Development of a Peer Support Network', *Australian Social Work*, vol. 50, no. 3, pp. 45–52

Howe, D. (1994) 'Modernity, Postmodernity and Social Work', *British Journal of Social Work*, vol. 24, pp. 513–32

Kingfisher, C.P. (1996) 'Women on Welfare: Conversational Sites of Aquiescence and Dissent', *Discourse and Society*, vol. 7, pp. 531–57

Kristeva, J. (1980), 'Woman Can Never Be Defined' (trans. M. R. Schuster) in E. Marks and I. De Courtivron (eds), *New French Feminisms: An Anthology*, University of Massachusetts Press, Amherst

——(1986) 'Women's Time' (trans. A. Jardine and H. Blake), in T. Moi (ed.), *The Kristeva Reader*, Columbia Press, New York, pp. 187–213

——(1991) *Strangers to Ourselves* (trans. Leon S. Roudiez), Columbia University Press, New York

Leonard, P. (1994) 'Knowledge/Power and Postmodernism: Implications for the Practice of a Critical Social Work Education', *Canadian Social Work Review*, vol. 11, no. 1, pp. 11–26

——(1995) 'Postmodernism, Socialism and Social Welfare', *Journal of Progressive Human Services*, vol. 6, no. 2, pp. 3–19

MacDonald, L. (1996) 'Dismantling the Movement: Feminism, Postmodernism and Politics', *Refractory Girl*, vol. 50, pp. 48–51

McHoul, A. and Grace, W. (1993) *A Foucault Primer: Discourse, Power and the Subject*, Melbourne University Press, Melbourne

McNay, M. (1992) 'Social Work and Power Relations: Towards a Framework for an Integrated Practice', in M. Langan and L. Day (eds), *Women, Oppression and Social Work: Issues in Anti-Discriminatory Practice*, London, Routledge

Middleman, R. and Goldberg, G. (1974) *Social Service Delivery: A Structural Approach to Social Work Practice*, Columbia University Press, New York

Moreau, M. (1979) 'A Structural Approach to Social Work Practice', *Canadian Journal of Social Work Education*, vol. 5, no.1, pp. 78–94

Parton, N. (1994) 'Problematics of Government, Postmodernity and Social Work', *British Journal of Social Work*, vol. 24, pp. 9–32

Pringle, R. (1995) 'Destabilising Patriarchy', in B. Caine and R. Pringle (eds), *Transitions: New Australian Feminism*, Allen & Unwin, Sydney

Ryburn, M. (1991) 'The Children Act: Power and Empowerment', *Adoption and Fostering*, vol. 15, no. 1, pp. 20–27

Sands, R. and Nuccio, K. (1992) 'Postmodern Feminist Theory and Social Work', *Social Work*, vol. 37, pp. 489–94

Scott, J.W. (1994) 'Deconstructing Equality-Versus-Difference: Or, the Uses of Poststructuralist Theory for Feminism', in S. Siedman (ed.), *The Postmodern Turn: New Perspectives on Social Theory*, Cambridge University Press, Cambridge

Tapper, M. (1993) 'Ressentiment and Power: Some Reflections on Feminist Practices', in P. Patton (ed.), *Nietzsche, Feminism and Political Theory*, Allen & Unwin, Sydney

Taylor-Gooby, P. (1993) 'Postmodernism and Social Policy: A Giant Leap Backwards', Social Policy Research Centre, Discussion Paper, no. 45, University of NSW, Kensington

Walby, S. (1992) 'Post-Post-Modernism? Theorising Social Complexity', in M. Barrett and A. Phillips (eds), *Destabilising Theory: Contemporary Feminist Debates*, Polity Press, Cambridge

Weedon, C. (1987) *Feminist Practice and Poststructuralist Theory*, Basil Blackwell, Oxford

West, C. (1995) 'Women's Competence in Conversation', *Discourse and Society*, vol. 3, 107–31

Wilson, E. (1977),'Women in the Community', in M. Mayo (ed.), *Women in the Community*, Routledge & Kegan Paul, London

Yeatman, A. (1993) 'Voice and the Representation of Difference', in A. Yeatman and S. Gunew (eds), *Feminism and the Politics of Difference*, Allen & Unwin, Sydney

——(1995) 'Interlocking Oppressions', in B. Caine and R. Pringle (eds), *Transitions: New Australian Feminisms*, Allen & Unwin, Sydney

——(1997) 'Feminism and Power', in M.L. Shanley and U. Narayan (eds), *Reconstructing Political Theory: Feminist Perspectives*, Polity Press, Oxford

Young, I.M. (1990) *Justice and the Politics of Difference*, Princeton University Press, Princeton, NJ

Community development and
a postmodernism of resistance
Mary Lane

I have a role in creating an atmosphere, or a way of being, that
promotes discussion and understanding. (Christley 1996: 96)

I could interpret Jon Christley's words as a postmodernist, yet
modernist, description of community development work. Whilst
being wary of thus slotting his work into my labels, I glimpse
some 'postmodernist' means—the use of a creative self, open and
flexible in promoting communication—combined with an agenda
which, in the spirit of modernism, prioritises certain enlightenment
values. As we shall see later in this chapter, the 'understanding'
sought is one which challenges prejudice and fear of difference,
and instead promotes respect and cooperation amongst people
from vastly different cultural backgrounds. His is not a statement
that 'anything goes' (as some say of postmodernity). Nor is it a
statement that 'I have a model of practice for all places and times'
(as some say of modernity).

In this chapter, I explore the problematic relationship between
postmodernism and modernism, arguing that there is no clear
divide between modernism/postmodernism and that ideas associated with some forms of postmodernism have much to contribute
to emancipatory practice in community development. In the spirit
of this book, we might refer to this as a 'critical postmodernist'
perspective towards practice—a proactive rather than reactive
postmodernism. Vignettes from community development in western and south-western Sydney will serve to develop this claim.

POSTMODERNISM

Postmodernism is a term used somewhat loosely to describe
cultural, social and political changes occurring in Western society.

A (modernist) culture, built over the last few centuries around forms of rationality, self-discipline and bourgeois values, is succumbing, it seems, to the effects of rapid technological and economic change. New cultural forms are emerging, challenging traditional values and ways of thinking. There is a realisation that the grand theories of modernity do not adequately explain the human condition and there is scepticism that the emancipatory ideals of modernity can ever be achieved—unemployment, poverty, ill-health, poor education, pollution and violence are still with us. Along with this loss of belief comes the triumph of a mass, commercial culture of consumerism and constant change. At least half of the world's population is now living in cities—a factor, it is argued, which contributes to separateness within massification (Rogers 1998: 23).

There is much debate as to whether these changes represent a crisis for modernity, that is, a complete break with traditions and beliefs of the past, or whether they are indicative of a transition towards another—perhaps a last—phase of modernity (Smart 1990; Best and Kellner 1991; Bauman 1992). Uncertainty about the extent and nature of the changes creates difficulties in understanding the concept of 'postmodernism'. There is a great deal of superficial and generalised writing and talking about it, particularly by those who send it up as just another 'fly by night' way of interpreting the 'present' (Grace 1998). Much of the discussion falls into the very trap that postmodernists point out as a weakness of modernist thinking—that is, the search for unitary definitions and the reduction under one label of complex clusters of thought (Wood 1997). There is not just one 'postmodernism' for us to agree with or reject; there are many aspects of a 'postmodern constellation'—just as there are, for instance, many 'socialisms' and 'feminisms'.

I find Smart's (1990) discussion of modernity and post-modernity helpful in clarifying meanings. Whilst noting that postmodernism is a 'polymorphous idea' (1990: 24), Smart also discusses a distinction between a 'postmodernism of reaction' and a 'postmodernism of resistance'. The former, he argues, repudiates modernity to affirm the status quo—eclecticism, populism and a principle of 'anything goes'. Smart identifies Jameson (1984) as a theorist of postmodernism who critiques such affirmation, arguing that postmodern cultural forms serve to reinforce the logic of consumer capitalism. Seen in this way, postmodernism is a conservative reaction: 'the cultural correlate of late, consumer or multi-national capitalism' (Smart 1990: 25).

A postmodernism of resistance, on the other hand, is about resisting the current status quo as well as deconstructing modernist traditions which cannot adequately explain and deal with present conditions. Referring particularly to Lyotard (1984, 1988), Smart develops an argument that this conception of postmodernism 'constitutes a counter-practice to official culture' (1990: 24). Critical, subversive and oppositional, this form of postmodernism thus has an affinity with some forms of modernism and with critical theory. It is this account of postmodernism which I find most useful for community development practice—a postmodernism of resistance, a 'critical postmodernism', which keeps some of the modern within the postmodern.

Keeping some of the modern within the postmodern is reminiscent of Habermas's (1987a, 1987b) defence of modernity as an unfinished project with, as yet, unfulfilled emancipatory potential. Habermas critiques much that is modern, particularly the notion of 'instrumental reason' which uncritically links means and ends. He argues instead for 'communicative rationality' and 'communicative action', grounded in mutual understanding, agreement and solidarity, and achieved through uncoerced communication.

The critical theory of Habermas, as with critical theory generally, is thus normative, allowing a standpoint for social action. This may seem to place critical theory in opposition to postmodernism. I am, however, inclined to the argument put by Best and Kellner (1991: 246–54) that there is much in common between postmodernism and critical theory, and much that is complementary. Both critique the status quo; both argue for the potential of language as the basis for critique and action. The differences are probably most obvious when we consider theories for action—the normative dimension of critical theory extending critique into theory-building about strategies for emancipatory social change. However, whilst postmodernists are wary of building blueprints for action, this does not necessarily rule out the possibility of pursuing social justice. Best and Kellner (1991: 250–51) note this point in their discussion of similarities in the politics of Habermas and Lyotard.

Acceptance of the potential complementarity of critical theory and a postmodernism of resistance opens the way for preserving a form of emancipatory practice amidst ever-changing contexts and the critiques of postmodernism. The forms of practice one might then expect would attempt to combine a concern with justice, such as how power and resources are distributed, with a resistance to developing generalised 'foundations' for practice. Strategies would reflect context, pluralism—and uncertainty.

With this exploration in mind, I now turn to some accounts of community development practice. I describe a way of working which many may argue is not new. I will deal with the question

of 'what's different?' in more detail later, only commenting here
that my point in telling these stories is to sharpen our analyses
and enrich our strategies through a postmodern reading. It is a
reading which calls into question structural analyses and blueprints for change based on 'universal' truth and value claims. My
reading, though, still carries with it the influence of critical
theorists such as Habermas, and those feminists who theorise
difference, and yet preserve some emancipatory values within their
critiques of modernity (Nicholson 1990; Barrett and Phillips
1992).

STORIES OF PRACTICE: LISTENING TO CONTEXT

The Sydney suburb of St Clair, as it was when the first community
development workers arrived in 1980, could well be described as
suffering from a 'postmodernist condition'—incomplete, isolated,
decentralised, fragmented and ahistorical. The government of New
South Wales, through its Land Commission, had offered 'the
world' to young home buyers settling in St Clair, a new housing
estate in outer western Sydney. Three years after development
began there was not a single service, but the government was still
rapidly selling off blocks of land. The population, already num-
bering over 3000, was growing by a thousand or more people
each year. Landcom acted like a private developer—maximising
profit from land selling, but doing nothing to provide the social
infrastructure.

Into this scene came three (all part-time) community development workers, funded by the federal government for an action
research project around childcare issues. Needing to learn about
the area and the people, to introduce themselves, to identify issues
of common concern and the potential for participation, they put
on their walking shoes and got on the track. With not even an
office, the car was a filing cabinet, and homes, 'parks', streets and
the pub in a neighbouring suburb were their working spaces. It
was summer and it was hot, but there were no trees to shade a
rest and a chat—they too had been bulldozed to make way for
the land dollar!

Many methods were used to meet residents, and to listen to
their stories about living in St Clair. A survey in the early months
involved knocking on every tenth door and interviewing over a
hundred people. As well, meetings were held in homes, and in
schools, baby clinics and other meeting places used by residents
outside the estate (no local community facilities having yet being
built).

Much was revealed in the ensuing dialogue with residents. The workers soon discovered that childcare issues were interlinked with multiple other problems requiring action, something which called for a broadened interpretation of their brief. They also discovered that preconceived definitions of need by local bureaucrats, government planners and a handful of vocal male resident leaders poorly matched those of the majority of residents. Priorities which had already been set included a tavern, a large sporting complex and facilities for organised sports. No plans were evident for neighbourhood and childcare centres, park development or the particular needs of girls and women. It was only resident action, prompted by the community development process that had revealed diverse interests and multiple voices, which forestalled the provision of costly, inappropriate services and led to provision more in tune with residents' immediate priorities.

The early contacting work was the means, then, for listening to and acting upon local knowledge—process-oriented work, networking people, ideas and resources—with the aim of changing the status quo. This approach, whilst traditionally well established in community development (Henderson and Thomas 1987; Lane 1990, 1992; Henry and Lane 1993), is out of fashion with decision-makers in product-oriented times of managed change. A postmodernist reading would, however, argue that such work—local, yet pluralistic—can lead to multiple opportunities for resistance to the status quo. 'Local' would be read not as a limited concept where all within some defined 'boundary' are assumed to have common interests, but as diverse, constantly changing networks of people who may negotiate common meanings in particular times and places. I further illustrate the point, using Kaylene Henry's story of starting her job in a public housing estate in Sydney's southwest (Henry 1993: 4–8). Here I look more closely at the worker's style.

Kaylene arrived in a more established area than St Clair. There had been a community worker before her, and there was an active community centre. Even so, Kaylene was well aware, from her reading, of the importance of a new worker gaining an understanding of 'community' as an initial step in community development practice. She anticipated spending her first month or so in the job preparing a profile of the area. She soon found that things were not so orderly; any ideas she had about a clear format for staging her work were shattered by the demands and interruptions of day-by-day activities in which she was expected to participate. 'This is how I learnt,' she says, 'that community profiles are not about collecting information to put in a document—they are about meeting people, learning as you are doing, and taking action as you go.'

She got a map of the area and walked around with several residents, marking landmarks and historical sites, land use, natural features, housing types, services, traffic and pedestrian routes, dangerous intersections, informal meeting places, areas of high vandalism. As she moved around the estate, she listened to local stories about history and about living in the area. To complement the mapping and the local stories, she collected any available statistics, contacted other service providers and community groups, doorknocked and took time to learn about her own organisation. Important information picked up in this contacting work was about power relations, including conflicts between community leaders. Kaylene found she had to be careful about who she aligned with—being cautious of paid workers with poor reputations in the estate, or of too readily being seen as joining the causes of particular community leaders. Describing what she learnt about getting started, Kaylene does not have a checklist for others about how to proceed, people to contact or things to look for, as so many 'how to' books do. Rather, she identifies four aspects which are more about personal style: being humble, visible, accessible and credible.

For our part, Kaylene's experience affirms that there are no ready-made solutions, and that best practice calls for developing, *as we go*, contextually appropriate purposes and strategies. Perhaps most importantly, the message is about creative use of self. Any packets of tricks which we carry as 'bunny rug woollies', from university or elsewhere, require critical reassessment within the 'chaos' of practice. Reading and experience alert us to possibilities, but we cannot uncritically transpose from one situation to another. Things are not always as we thought they would be—before we started!

RESISTING IMPOSED AGENDAS

These two vignettes reveal the discovery of many 'truths' and many stories which would remain hidden if the workers had *only* sat in an office, read reports, talked to policy-makers and examined statistical data—if it were available. A rich source of information is uncovered by acting on the question: 'What is the lived experience of the people with whom we are working?'

I repeat my earlier comments: that this approach, whilst familiar to many community development workers, bears retelling in the current climate of needs-based planning—that is, planning and consequently projects based on needs as identified by government and so-called 'experts'. Postmodernists would exhort us to resist the imposition of top-down agendas. Resistance is not always easy, however; it may mean sacrificing funding for projects and for workers. Following is a story about successful resistance in the face of such a threat—a story about the creative interpretation of the potentially narrow, conservative purposes of sponsors for broader, more transformative agendas.

Jon Christley worked in a medium density, public housing estate in southwestern Sydney, in an area which could only be termed 'ultra-multicultural'. Census figures identified 68 language groups and there was a constant influx of new arrivals, often from war-torn countries. Unemployment was endemic, and noise, water and air pollution high. The population included large numbers of children and adolescents; many residents were fearful of local youth gangs and crime was reportedly high. When Jon arrived in 1990, there was, however, a core of committed residents who had weathered these recurring problems since the estate was built in 1981 and who had a history of participation in local decision-making. A lot of local knowledge had been built up.

Jon worked in the area for five years. His painstaking, process-oriented approach to community development has been documented through video, audio-tape and written word (Lane and Vinson 1994; Christley and Lane 1992/3/4; Christley 1996). All describe an enabling, communicative, networking approach which, through participatory processes, sought to increase the decision-making power and the material and social resources of disadvantaged people.

Jon had been in the job a year when he was approached by a major insurance corporation seeking his assistance in undertaking a crime prevention project in the area—one of high cost saving to the corporation in terms of insurance claims! At first Jon and his employers (a large, local community development agency) were cautious about the project, not wanting to allow their community development work to be hijacked by an insurance company trying to reduce its costs. There was fear, too, that the corporation's understanding of community development was limited. Already the organisation had sponsored the setting up of neighbourhood watch projects in other areas which, in their terms, were a ready-made, cheap agenda for tackling theft and vandalism. Jon and many of the residents believed that these projects—based on control rather than prevention, on suspicion rather than trust, on spying on one's neighbour rather than developing neighbourliness, on single-objective rather than multiple-objective responses—were inconsistent with their community development purposes.

The situation was not straightforward, though. Crime and violence were also of much concern to residents. As well, the insurance group was offering a sizeable amount of money which could potentially be used for many badly needed community services and activities. At the risk of losing the money, Jon and his employers set out to transform the agenda. They entered a lengthy process of negotiation with the insurers, seeking to move the latter away from social control agendas driven by the immediacy of short-term costs towards a broad program of social development which, it was argued, would have longer lasting, positive outcomes for all concerned.

Negotiation required constant interpretation by Jon of the purposes and strategies of community development and of the need to have broad, flexible goals which would be responsive to constantly changing circumstances and would be developed with the extensive involvement of local residents.

Jon also needed to challenge, to deconstruct, prevailing theories of how to deal with violence and crime. The 1980s and 1990s have seen emphasis on inherency theories of crime and violence. Control and retribution have been the favoured strategic responses, rather than rehabilitation and prevention through social development. Consequently, there has been a move towards more gaols, tougher punishments and focused interventions—for example, regulating drinking in night clubs and public places (Homel et al. 1992; Homel et al. 1994); enclosing housing developments (Morgan 1994); changing the design of public spaces (Sarkissian et al. 1992); and even genetic screening (Wayt Gibbs 1995)! In spite of some significant studies in the United States, The Netherlands and France (Milton Eisenhower Foundation 1990) and some interesting projects and thoughtful theorists in Australia (Hiller 1995; White and Sutton 1995), it has been difficult to argue for social development as a means of tackling crime and violence.

In this case, however, an argument for contextually sensitive social development was successful. The corporation offered $80 000 over three years for projects which it agreed would be identified by residents themselves through a community development process. Jon and his employing agency agreed to take the project on, as long as it was seen as part of, not separate from, the broad program of community development and commitment to change that he and the residents were already undertaking. In this way, they would not be lackeys of the insurance company and recognition was given to the interconnectedness of issues, problems and responses.

It is not my purpose here to elaborate upon the details of the project and its outcomes; rather, I am highlighting a style of practice which brings radical critique and a postmodernist scepticism to bear upon dominant explanations and agendas developed from 'on high'.

HOLDING ON TO OUR ETHICS: DIFFERENCE AND 'COMMUNITY'

Being responders to context rather than imposers of already established formulae for action need not mean working in an ethical vacuum of an 'anything goes' postmodernism where all views must be accepted as having equal value. We are not forced to work with people whose causes we oppose, and who do not respect our values or those of others—we too, have the right of speech and the right of refusal. Whilst we cannot assume a unitary set of ethics about which there is universal agreement, we can hold on to our personal ethics. This point is well demonstrated in the following two accounts of anti-racist practice in southwest Sydney.

The location for the first is a broadacre housing development area, again with a very ethnically diverse population. Linda Livingstone was the first community development worker to be based in the estate. She worked from a neighbourhood centre, and when she arrived only a few people from non-English speaking backgrounds were involved with the centre which was dominated by 'Anglo' Australians. In a story about her work, Linda explains how she set out to increase the participation of non-English speaking people in community activities and local decision-making (Livingstone 1993: 24–26). For these purposes, her strategies were similar to those of the workers in the vignettes above—a great deal of face-to-face personal contact. As she says: 'You must constantly look at your community first, go out to them, learn from them; you just cannot read your textbook and throw yourself into it' (1993: 24).

Linda soon encountered racism, which she dealt with in several ways. In discussions between people, she openly confronted what she considered to be racist remarks and behaviour, by labelling it and acting as 'adjudicator'. She also dealt with racism in what she called 'more subtle ways', taking advantage of everyday activities to increase communication between people (1993: 25–26):

> One way is to expose people to working with people from other cultures; for instance, leaving one of the non-English speaking

women to work with one of the Anglo-Australian women in the
kitchen. Or picking different people up in my car, where they have
to share the backseat and participate in everyday conversation.
They soon realise they have a lot of similarities.

Linda's work reveals a process of critical reflection, whereby she
developed theories for practice to suit the context, rather than the
textbook. We could liken her approach to that of a postmodernism
of resistance. The workers' values are clear; there is no resem-
blance to a postmodernism of 'whatever'.

Jon Christley, whose work I have already referred to above,
used somewhat similar approaches. He confronted racism when it
occurred overtly in interpersonal relationships and he also worked
on a broader front, through community development processes,
to promote inter-cultural understanding and to challenge institutional racism (Christley 1996: 95–96). He describes the growth of
understanding, and respect for difference, as a long process promoted by people doing things together, listening to each other and
realising they have issues in common. Whilst non-directive, his
approach is clearly purposeful rather than rehabilitation and
prevention through social development, and reflects his values
(anti-racist, pro-mutual respect) (1996: 95–96):

> As the community worker, I am the person who may try and help
> them interpret each other, or improve that communication. My
> role is to facilitate the getting together. I have a role in creating
> an atmosphere, or a way of being that promotes discussion and
> understanding.

In a postmodern world of difference, holding on to personal
ethics is one thing, but can there ever be enough agreement about
values and purposes to pursue social action aimed at challenging
inequalities and oppression? Herein lies the seed of the difference
between critical theory and extreme postmodernism: for the latter,
the celebration of difference takes precedence over normative goals
and the question of what sort of society we should seek. Extreme
postmodernism implies that 'community' is dead—and with it,
community development.

Barbara Epstein (1995) notes a similar point. In a discussion
of the influence of radical poststructuralism upon feminism, she
argues that poststructuralism (a term she seems to use synony-
mously with postmodernism) is 'a dead end' for progressive
thought or social change (1995: 83–84). She is one of many
expressing the fear that a postmodern celebration of diversity and
difference will work against the development of common cause

amongst vulnerable groups, and will lead to inequalities (Brodribb 1992; Taylor-Gooby 1994).

Whilst Epstein and Brodribb express these fears, other feminists, though recognising the potential dilemma, have theorised difference *and* argued for engagement in political action to further the causes of women as a whole (Nicholson 1990; Barrett and Phillips 1992; Sands and Nuccio 1992). The notion of a clear divide between modern/postmodern is deconstructed.

'Community' is, however, fragile in postmodern terms, not only because of emphasis on difference, but because meaning and connection are linguistically, rather than structurally, understood. Common purpose may be found, though, through 'the maximisation of speech' (Erasaari 1985: 19), whereby we interpret and present our 'worlds' of meaning to one another (Howe 1994; Pardeck et al. 1994; Lane 1997). As we have seen, this was the very task of the community development workers in the stories. Community is developed through a feast of communication in which people are respected and encouraged to express their views. Truth and value claims are negotiated in particular places, times and contexts.

A postmodernist understanding of community, fragile and temporary as it is, can also be emancipatory. Emphasis on a subjective, negotiated community, rather than belief in community as an objective reality (which then imposes identity upon people), allows people to construct their own identity and promotes the inclusion of previously excluded voices in decision-making. The tensions and conflicts associated with recognition of diverse values and interests are then not denied, but rather acknowledged and made part of the negotiating process. It is difficult, painstaking work, but as community development workers have found, such work increases the chances of finding common meanings, even where there has been much conflict (Mahtani 1996: 51–52). The search for common meaning lives with dissent, and grows from it, rather than subduing it.

POSTMODERNISM AND COMMUNITY DEVELOPMENT: BRING ON THE ARTIST!

My reluctance to impose labels upon practice prevents me from saying that the stories I have used are examples of 'critical postmodernism' in practice. Perhaps, though, the vignettes could be seen to describe a way of doing things which is consistent with ideas associated with critical theory and with a postmodernism of resistance. The *rationale* for the work is to challenge injustices and seek changes which will benefit disadvantaged groups of people. The *approach* reflects a postmodernist openness and uncertainty; responsiveness to context; resistance to imposed agendas and values; respect for diversity and celebration of difference; and rejection of arrogant professionalism which privileges the skills and knowledge of a few over lived experience. Questioning, listening, encouraging, responding, the worker is a promoter of speech, an interpreter of meanings and a networker of ideas and people.

Does this offer a new approach to community development, or is it a statement, in different language, of a way of practising which has been around for a long while? Perhaps it is the latter, but we still need to bring it into focus to argue its relevance for the present. In doing so, we might also recall another 'oldie goldie'—the concept of the 'animateur', referred to by Elphick many years ago in his discussion of community arts and community development (Elphick 1980).

The cultural animateur seeks change through relationship-building, encouraging people to meet, to form networks and to express their needs, desires and aspirations through creative forms of expression. Drawing on Hurstel (1974: 100), Elphick describes the function of the animateur as:

> breaking with former ossified functions and unsuitable professional structures; it introduces new practices and new methods marked by a concern for democracy, for inter-personal relationships, for popular expression. The animateur is 'a creator of exchanges, forms and contradictions'.

The purposes, functions and processes of the animateur seem just as appropriately to describe the contextually responsive, network-building community development referred to earlier. Highlighted is community development as an art.

THE PROBLEM IS, THOUGH, THAT THIS WAY OF WORKING IS RARELY PRACTISED TODAY

Community development is under siege as a process-oriented, contextually sensitive means of promoting participation in civil society and politics. Agendas are handed down with funding packages; accountability is to funders rather than to those who may be affected by interventions; and emphasis is on predefined goals rather than on accounts of lived experience. The worker might well be described as a manager, rather than an enabler.

We begin to see that the vignettes referred to earlier are

examples of resistance, of a counter-practice, and that the way of working they describe resembles that of an artist. If we seek to challenge the official culture, we need to bring these ways into focus again and critique them, as we have, in the light of the present. A postmodern reading prompts us to question everything, but also opens up the possibility of multiple explanations and multiple strategies.

The challenges inspired by postmodernism can lead us to ever-more creative practice. In the last half of the twentieth century, we have built some solid practice castles from modernity. I believe it is time to move on from those ageing, modernist structures, and their generalised 'models', 'competencies' and narrow 'scientific' ways of knowing. It is time to immerse our-selves in ever-changing networks and domains. We are uncertain about many things but we have memory, personal ethics and the magic of speech. We are confident in our ability to speak, to listen and interpret, to encourage subdued voices. We are confident that community, though fragile, is possible.

And with us are Lyotard, Habermas and those very helpful feminists who encourage us to theorise difference whilst yet retain-ing commitment to justice and social action. Resistance, uncertainty and difference with justice—a tricky, but not impos-sible, combination for postmodern times. Bring on the artist . . .

REFERENCES

Barrett, M. and Phillips, A. (eds) (1992) *Destabilizing Theory: Contemporary Feminist Debates*, Polity Press, Cambridge

Bauman, Z. (1992) *Intimations of Postmodernity*, Routledge, London and New York

Best, S. and Kellner, D. (1991) *Postmodern Theory: Critical Interrogations*, Macmillan, Basingstoke

Brodribb, S. (1992) *Nothing Mat(t)ers: A Feminist Critique of Postmodern-ism*, Spinifex Press, Melbourne

Christley, J. (1996) 'Jon Christley's Story', in J. Christley and M. Lane (eds), *In This Place: Stories of Villawood*, Christley Lane Publications, Castle Hill

Christley, J. and Lane, M. (1992/3/4) Villawood Interviews, unpublished audio-tapes

Elphick, C. (1980) 'Community Arts and Community Development: Socio-Cultural Animation', in P. Henderson, D. Jones and D.N. Thomas (eds), *The Boundaries of Change in Community Work*, George Allen & Unwin, London, pp. 98–109

Epstein, B. (1995) 'Why Post-structuralism is a Dead End for Progressive Thought', *Socialist Review*, vol. 25, no. 2, pp. 83–119

Erasaari, R. (1985) The New Social State, paper presented to the Fourth International Conference on the Comparative Historical and Critical Analysis of Bureaucracy: 'Bureaucracy and Culture', Simon Fraser University, Burnaby/Vancouver, available as a New Waverley Paper

Grace, D. (1998) 'A Strange Outbreak of Rocks in the Head', *The Sydney Morning Herald*, 21 January, p. 13

Habermas, J. (1987a) *The Theory of Communicative Action* (T. McCarthy trans.), Polity Press, Cambridge

——(1987b) *The Philosophical Discourse of Modernity: Twelve Lectures* (Frederick Lawrence, trans.), MIT Press, Cambridge, Mass.

Henderson, P. and Thomas, D.N. (1987) *Skills in Neighbourhood Work*, 2nd edn, Unwin Hyman, London

Henry, K. (1993) 'Contacting', in K. Henry and M. Lane (eds), *Once Upon a Time . . . Stories About Community Work*, Local Community Services Association, Surry Hills, NSW, pp. 4–8

Henry, K. and Lane, M. (1993) *Once Upon a Time . . . Stories About Community Work*, Local Community Services Association, Surry Hills, NSW

Hiller, A. (1995) 'Developments in Community Policing—Beat Policing Pilot Projects in Queensland', *Australian Police Journal*, June, pp. 105–10.

Homel, R., Hauritz, M., Wortley, R., Clark, J. and Carvolth, R. (1994) *The Impact of the Surfers Paradise Safety Action Project: Key Findings of the Evaluation*, Centre for Crime Policy and Public Safety, School of Justice Administration, Griffith University, Brisbane

Homel, R., Tomsen, S. and Thommeny, J. (1992) 'Public Drinking and Violence: Not Just an Alcohol Problem', *The Journal of Drug Issues*, vol. 22, no. 3, pp. 679–97

Howe, D. (1994) 'Modernity, Postmodernity and Social Work', *British Journal of Social Work*, vol. 24, no. 5, pp. 513–32

Hurstel, J. (1974) *Training of Animateurs*, Strasbourg, Council of Europe

Jameson, F. (1984) 'Postmodernism or the Cultural Logic of Late Capitalism', *New Left Review*, no. 146, pp. 53–92

Lane, M. (1990) 'Community Work with Immigrant Groups', *Australian Social Work*, vol. 43, no. 3, pp. 33–38

——(1992) 'Community Work, Social Change and Women', in J. Petruchenia and R. Thorpe (eds), *Social Change and Social Welfare Practice*, Hale and Iremonger, Sydney, pp. 166–79

——(1997) 'Community Work, Social Work: Green and Postmodern?', *British Journal of Social Work*, vol. 27, no. 3, pp. 319–41

Lane, M. and Vinson, T. (1994) *Community Development and Crime: The RISE Project*, School of Social Work, University of New South Wales; and Department of Social Work, Social Policy and Sociology, University of Sydney, a video tape.

Livingstone, L. (1993) 'Anti-racist Practice', in K. Henry and M. Lane (eds),

Once Upon a Time . . . Stories About Community Work, Local Community Services Association, Surry Hills, NSW, pp. 23–26

Lyotard, J.F. (1984) *The Postmodern Condition: A Report on Knowledge*, Geoff Bennington and Brian Massumi (trans.), Manchester University Press, Manchester

——(1988) 'An Interview', *Theory, Culture and Society*, vol. 5, nos 2–3, pp. 277–310

Mahtani, S. (1996) 'Sundar Mahtani's Story', in J. Christley and M. Lane (eds), *In This Place: Stories of Villawood*, Christley Lane Publications, Castle Hill, pp. 39–52

Milton Eisenhower Foundation (1990) *Youth Investment and Community Reconstruction: Street Lessons on Drugs and Crime for the Nineties*, A Tenth Anniversary Report, Milton Eisenhower Foundation, USA

Morgan, G. (1994) 'Acts of Enclosure: Crime and Defensible Space in Contemporary Cities', in G. Gibson and S. Watson (eds), *Metropolis Now*, Pluto Press, Melbourne, pp. 78–90

Nicholson, L. (ed.) (1990) *Feminism/Postmodernism*, Routledge, New York

Pardeck, J.T., Murphy, J.W. and Min Choi, J. (1994) 'Some Implications of Postmodernism for Social Work', *Social Work*, vol. 39, no. 4, pp. 343–46

Rogers, R. (1998) 'City Limits', *The Australian Magazine*, 7–8 February, pp. 23–26

Sarkissian, W. (ed.) with Whitzman, C., Rosier, L. and Llewellyn, J. (1992) *Safe as Houses: Proceedings of a Griffith University Workshop on Crime Prevention Through Environmental Design*, Research and Policy Paper No. 2, Centre for Crime Policy and Public Safety, School of Justice Administration, Griffith University, Brisbane

Sands, R.G. and Nuccio, K. (1992) 'Postmodern Feminist Theory and Social Work', *Social Work*, vol. 37, no. 6, pp. 489–94

Smart, B. (1990) 'Modernity, Postmodernity and the Present' in B.S. Turner (ed.), *Theories of Modernity and Postmodernity* Sage, London and Newbury Park, Cal.

Taylor-Gooby, P. (1994) 'Postmodernism and Social Policy: A Great Leap Backwards?', *Journal of Social Policy*, vol. 23, no. 3, pp. 385–404

Wayt Gibbs, W. (1995) 'Seeking the Criminal Element', *Scientific American*, March, pp. 76–83

White, R. and Sutton, A. (1995) 'Crime Prevention, Urban Space and Social Exclusion', *The Australian and New Zealand Journal of Sociology*, vol. 31, no. 1, pp. 82–99

Wood, C. (1997) 'To Know or Not to Know: A Critique of Postmodernism in Social Work Practice', *Australian Social Work*, vol. 50, no. 3, pp. 21–27

10 Empowerment: The modernist social work concept *par excellence*
Stephen Parker, Jan Fook and Bob Pease

How do we reconceptualise empowerment from a postmodern perspective? This chapter is concerned with addressing this question. First we will look briefly at modernist notions of power and empowerment, and examine the issues which make these problematic. Next we will review some of the major ways in which postmodern perspectives can inform direct practice, and how these may apply to the idea of empowerment. Finally, we will reformulate the concept of empowerment from these perspectives.

MODERNIST NOTIONS OF EMPOWERMENT

Modernist liberal and socialist traditions, with their themes of progress and emancipation, have been able to provide social workers with a sense of broader purpose, so that daily practice could be interpreted and connected with these overriding goals. However, the daily inequalities and injustices confronted by social workers still exist. Additionally, although these modern conceptualisations of power have supported emancipatory ideals, they have also become confused with the 'normalising power' of modern society as conceptualised by Foucault (1980). By 'normalising power', Foucault means the mechanisms by which individuals conform to the regulatory processes of government and society.

The result of this confusion has been reflected in the difficulty faced by social workers in trying to define and apply the concept of empowerment. One of the paradoxes of empowerment is that it has both liberatory and regulatory potential (Baistow 1994/95: 35). According to Baistow, empowerment discourses imply that the power is actually power over oneself, not others. Furthermore, they promote a type of individualised non-reflexive responsibility—empowerment is done *to* you *by* others, or done *by* you *to* others (1994/95: 38–39). In this sense, it is professionals who have colonised empowerment and this, by definition, means that empowerment is taken out of the hands of those who are being empowered. Hoy (1986), however, makes the point that both empowered and disempowered groups (the dominated and dominating) are part of the network of power relations (1986: 134). With these apparent contradictions in mind, are our current modern notions of emancipation reasonable and achievable?

THE DILEMMA OF DIFFERENCE

Minow (1985) illustrates that one of the paradoxes of empowerment is that it can have disempowering functions. There is a dilemma in identifying a particular group in dire need of resources, and then seeking to provide the identified group with those resources, only to find that membership of that group has become stigmatised. The 'difference dilemma' for service providers, therefore, are how is it possible to identify and provide services to a group without, at the same time, labelling and stigmatising that group?

The 'dilemma of difference' provides a good way of conceptualising some of the problems faced by social workers in their attempts to apply the concept of empowerment in their practice. Social workers could be understood as being in a paradoxical position in which the very work they are seeking to do in order to empower people may at the same time be interpreted as damaging, or even disempowering. There is, perhaps, something in the modernist approach to empowerment which contributes to, rather than avoids, the 'dilemma of difference'.

If the modernist perspective, with its scientific basis and rationalist approach, is about following a process such as examining an aspect or area of practice, identifying a problem or problems, categorising the people involved, and then targeting those people for a provision of service, this type of activity could be argued to be stigmatising—to be contributing to a 'difference dilemma'. The conceptions of power associated with the 'liberal' and 'socialist' traditions—that is, individually focused and with a powerful/powerless dichotomy respectively—again appear to contribute to, rather than seek to avoid, the 'difference dilemma'.

Foucault's conception of the 'normalising power' in modern

society best expresses the underlying process that results in the 'dilemma of difference'. Normalising power in modern society is about separating people from each other, labelling some as deviants to be subjected to the carceral network—a network which has extended to take in the whole of society (Foucault 1977).

Social workers experience the paradox inherent in the 'difference dilemma' by relying upon modernist conceptions of power when confronting the 'normalising power' in modern society. We would argue that the problems social workers have experienced in defining and applying the concept of empowerment reflect this underlying problem of their conception of power. Facing examples of inequality and injustice in their work, social workers have promoted the importance of empowerment. However, social workers' underlying conception of power has, we would argue, contributed to paradoxical dilemmas in their practice, such as the 'dilemma of difference'. The radical hope for emancipation attached to these modernist conceptions of empowerment has not been matched by the critical insight of these conceptions.

Minow (1985) suggests a way out of the difference dilemma. She argues that we need to re-immerse ourselves in the dilemma, not avoid it, in order to yield a more vivid understanding, and that what we are hoping for is not a solution but a more productive struggle. This involves rethinking the concept of 'difference'. Rather than focusing on difference or ignoring it, we need to locate it in the relationship rather than in the person or group called 'different'. This may permit a new stance towards the problem of stigma by acknowledging difference without turning it into the 'other' (1985: 202–206).

In describing the process which results in the 'dilemma of difference', Minow could equally be describing the process of 'normalising power' in modern society, reflecting Foucault's conception of power. Minow's rethinking of 'difference' is an example of a 'postmodern perspective'—a perspective which, while not seeking to resolve the various problems facing contemporary society, rather recasts the problems so as to suggest a way out of the dilemmas confronted with the use of a modernist approach.

POSTMODERN PERSPECTIVES AND SOCIAL WORK PRACTICE

Drawing upon those writers who have considered the impact of postmodernism upon social work practice, we will look at the concept of empowerment from a postmodern perspective. Parton (1994: 94), for example, argues that social work can be seen as providing a compromise between the liberal vision of unhindered private philanthropy and the socialist vision of the all-pervasive state which would take responsibility for everyone's needs and hence undermine the responsibility and role of the family (1994: 94).

In considering modernist social work's use of the concept of empowerment, it is easy to see how, given Parton's understanding of the emergence of modern social work, the concept of empowerment reflects aspects of both the liberal and socialist traditions.

Given that postmodernity is characterised by fragmentation, for Parton the implication for social work practice is that 'the pursuit of an ideal consensus is seen as misguided'. What is needed, therefore, is a more accepting attitude towards contingency and particularly the various 'language games'. A primary goal of social work is to try to enhance intelligibility between different cultures. The implication for practice, therefore, is not to eliminate contingency, but to create the conditions that will enable people to exercise self-determination in the face of contingency (1994: 110).

For Parton, accepting that we live in and with contingency does not represent a loss, for the promise of certainty was from the outset unrealisable. It is the pursuit of self-determination in cooperation with others that allows us to transform our contingency into destiny (1994: 110).

Pardek et al. (1994: 115) point to the importance of language in a postmodern perspective. Instead of being described as a tool that merely points to objects, language is understood to mediate thoroughly everything that is known. Reality is thus not obtrusive, but embedded within interpretation, and emerges from the language and associated constructed behaviour of people. Facts are thus local or regional. The implication for social work practice is that social workers should strive for 'communicative competence', rather than gathering 'objective' data, which may have limited cultural relevance (Pardeck et al. 1994: 116).

What is new about this postmodern approach is that clients are not merely consulted—through the use of individualised treatment plans, for instance—but supply the interpretive framework that is necessary for determining a proper intervention or a successful treatment strategy. This is truly client-centred intervention (Pardeck et al. 1994: 120). This client-centredness and contextualisation potentially undermine the traditional hierarchy in that status-based or absolute truth claims are subverted, and traditional expertise can be challenged. The ability to create locally appropriate realities (1994: 128) becomes possible.

POSTMODERN PERSPECTIVES AND EMPOWERMENT

In the foregoing discussion, both Parton and Pardek et al. identify an emancipatory aspect to a postmodern approach to social work practice. Given this emancipatory objective, what are the implications for the concept of empowerment?

Healy and Fook (1994) argue that Foucault's conceptualisation of power ('power is exercised, not possessed') is potentially useful for social workers who are interested in empowerment and the achievement of social justice ends (1994: 25). The emphasis, however, is on *potential*, since it should be noted that Foucault's analysis of power may be used equally as well to empower the more powerful, as well as the less powerful groups. This understanding of the limitations and potential for empowerment is integral to a postmodern perspective, because emancipation and repression are not inherent within specific discourses. It is not inevitable that an emancipatory discourse will automatically lead to emancipatory practices (Healy and Fook 1994: 25–26).

The emancipatory possibilities that Healy and Fook (1994) identify in relation to Foucault's conception of power and his analysis of power relations in society are presented in three interrelated aspects. First, in order to develop strategies to contest current dominant discourses and practices, we clearly need to understand the many ways in which discourses interrelate with other discourses, and with the power relationships which both produce and are produced by the discourses (1994: 27). Second, a multifaceted analysis, such as Foucault's, suggests many possible points of choice and resistance. Finally, as this analysis recognises the presence of contradictions, uncertainty and changeability (1994: 27), it might better be able to deal with the specific practice dilemmas faced by social workers.

Another dilemma raised by Weedon (1987) is that of complicity with oppression (cited in Healy and Fook 1994: 27). This dilemma concerns how and why people may be said to participate in their own oppression. The benefit of the analysis of power relations suggested by Foucault, in respect of complicity with oppression, is that, given various local interpretations of the person's situation, this contextualising may determine whether the person is empowered or not in respect of the power relations which affect him or her. What may be empowering in one setting may not be empowering in another.

This seeming paradox in regard to the understanding and application of the concept of empowerment is raised by Baistow, as discussed earlier, in terms of the regulatory as well as liberatory implications of the empowerment discourse (1994/95: 34).

The paradoxes that Baistow describes in the use of the concept of empowerment all reflect the problems that arise for the use of empowerment when modern conceptions of power (as a basis for empowerment) face the power of normalising society. Baistow discusses the example of power being removed from professionals and restored to ordinary citizens (1994/95: 38). The underlying conception of power is modern—that is, power as a possession, empowerment as power shifting from the powerless to the powerful.

As Baistow demonstrates, the irony is that professionals are increasingly seen to be central to the process of empowerment, rather than being rendered less powerful by it (1994: 39). Modernist conceptions of empowerment do not appear to be able to explain this contradictory phenomenon. Empowerment can thus give voice to the experience of powerlessness, but the real question is whether it can survive as a construct with critical potential while it remains a professional tool (1994/95: 45).

Can postmodern perspectives assist in developing a concept of critical empowerment which is used by people to empower themselves according to differing situations? This question states the position of social workers who wish to hold on to the radical hope for emancipation connected to the concept of empowerment, yet recognise the lack of critical insight or critical potential associated with the use of the concept. When Baistow discusses the paradox of the liberatory and regulatory aspects connected to the concept of empowerment, she is reaffirming the radical hope of empowerment in the face of the normalising, regulatory power in society. To confront this paradox requires rethinking empowerment from a postmodern critical perspective.

A postmodern critical concept of empowerment, however, may mean at the very least reconsidering social work's radical hope for empowerment. The work of Lather (1991) is helpful in fleshing out the ways in which discourses may or may not be emancipatory. In discussing the role of intellectuals in social change, she emphasises the importance of self-reflexivity in those who speak for and objectify others, reminding us that we contribute to dominance in spite of our liberatory intentions (1991: 15). Lather's description of the intellectual who both objectifies and speaks for others can be applied appropriately to the social worker who seeks to empower others through a process of labelling, targeting and providing a service.

CONSTRUCTING A POSTMODERN CONCEPTION OF EMPOWERMENT

If the postmodern perspective allows space to conceptualise how our own practice may contribute to our dominance in spite of our liberatory intentions, what does this mean for a postmodern conception of empowerment?

We would argue that this first requires being conscious of how the very defining of power constructs not only how power is understood, but can also either make clear or obscure modern expressions of power. The very act of conceiving power is part of the struggle over power (Hoy 1986: 144). Thus it is important to construct new conceptions of power relations. It is also imperative to recognise and resist expressions of normalising power in society wherever and whenever this may be possible.

The postmodern process of empowerment is not simply about defining away problems, but instead being open to alternative interpretations of situations through developing communicative competence. Strategies for practice which may emerge from this communication, if they are to challenge dominant discourses and practices, will require an understanding of how power relationships both produce and are produced by discourses (Healy and Fook 1994: 27).

It is our belief that social workers are well placed to take up the challenge of rethinking their practice understandings from a postmodern perspective because the very emergence of modernist social work can be interpreted as a 'postmodern-like' phenomena. By this we mean that modernist social work may be thought of as operating in the space between many of the 'incommensurates' of modern society—that is, between the public and the private and the government and the family. Modernist social work represents a compromise between the liberal vision and the socialist vision (Parton 1994: 94) and between what is considered 'safe' and 'dangerous' in society.

The uncertainty or uneasiness that may come with the postmodern perspective may actually be welcomed by many social workers, who may feel that such understandings and interpretations may, to a great extent, capture their experience of practising contemporary social work under the conditions of postmodernity.

REFERENCES

Baistow, K. (1994/95) 'Liberation or Regulation? Some Paradoxes of Empowerment', *Critical Social Policy*, no. 42 (Winter) pp. 34–46

Berman, M. (1982) *All that is Solid Melts into Air,* Verso, London

Dreyfus, H. and Rabinow, P. (1982) *Michel Foucault: Beyond Structuralism and Hermenuetics,* University of Chicago Press, Chicago

Foucault, M. (1977) *Discipline and Punish,* Allan Lane, London

——(1980) *Power/Knowledge: Selected Interviews and Other Writings 1972–1977,* Pantheon Books, New York

Healy, B. and Fook, J. (1994) 'Reinventing Social Work', in J. Ife (ed.), *Advances in Social Work and Welfare Education,* University of Western Australia, Perth

Hoy, D.C. (ed.) (1986) *Foucault: A Critical Reader,* Basil Blackwell, Oxford

Lather, P. (1991) *Getting Smart: Feminist Research and Pedagogy with/in the Postmodern,* Routledge, New York

Minow, M. (1985) 'Learning to Live with the Dilemma of Difference: Bilingual and Special Education', *Law and Contemporary Problems,* vol. 18, no. 2, pp. 157–211

Oliver, J. and Huxley, P. (1994) 'Editorial', *Social Work and Social Sciences Review,* vol. 8, no. 2, pp. 91–92

Pardeck, J.T., Murphy, J.W. and Min Choi, J. (1994) 'Some Implications of Postmodernism for Social Work', *Social Work,* vol. 39, no. 4, pp. 343–46

Parton, N. (1994) 'The Nature of Social Work Under the Conditions of (Post)Modernity', *Social Work and Social Sciences Review,* vol. 5, no. 2, pp. 93–112

Weedon, C. (1987) *Feminist Practice and Poststructuralist Theory,* Basil Blackwell, Oxford

PART IV
Reconstructing social work education

Postmodernism and the
teaching and practice of
interpersonal skills
*Helen Jessup and
Steve Rogerson*

INTRODUCTION

Interpersonal communication is the primary medium for the practice of social work. Yet social work has long borrowed the tools of other disciplines, specifically psychology, in the arena of micro skills, producing a dissonance for practitioners. Our belief is that social work is a separate discipline and as such requires a specific form of interpersonal communication practice as a vehicle for its particular concern: the interface between the personal and sociostructural.

We have designed a process for both teaching and practising interpersonal communication which produces an educational rather than a therapeutic landscape. This offers critical emancipatory skills which express contemporary postmodernist ideas. As a device for assisting access to some of these ideas, we have invented an imaginary respondent to ask us questions about our approach. This enables us to ground our explanations in an more accessible conversational style and breaks the monological tone of one voice.

WHY DEVELOP A POSTMODERN APPROACH TO TEACHING AND PRACTISING INTERPERSONAL COMMUNICATION SKILLS?

As qualified social workers and teachers of welfare workers, our experience was that the training courses on which we taught, and had ourselves been taught, included a critical structuralist approach to practice. Yet the teaching and practice of interpersonal communication (micro-skills) produced a dichotomy because they were not integrated with this critical approach. Students and teachers were often confused, being taught incongruent theoretical approaches which resulted in the situation that practitioners either 'did' social change or they 'do' interpersonal work.

We say this because interpersonal communication appears to represent a void in the development of a social work practice which is concerned with dismantling those forms of power relations which place individuals, groups, communities—whole cultures—in situations of oppression and distress. As social workers, we were well versed in the so-called 'radical' practice of social work, including community work, advocacy and political action. Yet casework, including interpersonal communication, was regarded as suspect by many because it remained determined by a therapeutic explanation of human difficulty grounded in humanistic ideas.

In other words, what distinguishes social work from other corollary disciplines—psychology, psychiatry, even primary health care—was omitted from interpersonal communication. On the one hand, we were teaching students critical social change through political practice—locating individual difficulty within a sociostructural context—with modules such as 'Social and Economic Issues' and 'Social Processes'. Yet, at the same time, students would be taught to interview a 'client' or other interviewee by listening, following, responding empathically and so forth. They would explore problems, current/past relationships, childhood, behavioural patterns, motivation, intent, responsibility, honesty. We were teaching technical skills within humanist principles, without reference to any political context. Students themselves identified this dissonance. At that stage, we did not have the means to apply comparative political analysis to interpersonal communication skills theorists and their practice skills, as we did with other aspects of the course.

The risk in teaching in that way was to produce a social work response to oppressive social structures which remained largely a theoretical exercise, since the practice of critical strategies relied on the most basic of skills (talking to one another). These 'different' modes of practice were located within paradoxical theories of social change. We were searching for new knowledge which would bridge this divide.

WHAT DOES POSTMODERNISM OFFER?

Fundamentally, the poststructuralism of Foucault and the educational strategy of Freire provide the theoretical framework for teaching and practising critical emancipatory interpersonal communication skills. Foucault's poststructuralism is particularly useful because it offers a political approach to social construction rather than the often nihilistic deconstruction of some other postmodernist writers. This distinction between poststructuralism and postmodernism is important. Peters (1995: 10) reminds us about the latter that:

> postmodernism signifies a change in people's relation to . . . meaning . . . the conditions of existence of meaning(s) can no longer be taken for granted or blithely assumed. Meaning must be understood as implicated in power relations . . . meaning/knowledge/truth has lost its innocence and so have we.

To borrow a concept of Calinescu (1987), poststructuralism can be conceptualised as a 'face' of postmodernism. It has grown out of the ideas and practices of postmodernism, but deals with the implications of language as a producer of the social and cultural world. Its focus is around disclosing the implications of cultural and social discourse as a production of the interaction of people whose very subjectivity is a product of that discourse. Most importantly, it is a site for realising the critical potential for change within the postmodern world. Lonsdale (1991: 11) comments:

> Poststructuralism can be understood as that theoretical 'stream' within the broader umbrella of postmodernism which radically subverts and problematises taken for granted assumptions about language.

Poststructuralism considers language to be the producer of meaning. This is in contradistinction to the notion which has dominated previous interpersonal communication theory and practice: that language is a reflector of reality.

LANGUAGE IS IMPORTANT HERE?

The interpersonal communication processes we use as social beings primarily involve language in its many forms. Amongst poststructural theorists, language is a collective concern. As Chris Weedon (1987: 21) puts it:

> Language is the place where actual and possible forms of social organisation and their likely social and political consequences are defined and contested. Yet it is also the place where our sense of ourselves, or subjectivity, is constructed.

Immediately, then, the site for change appears in the many forms of language and their 'signified' meanings. This suggests a powerful strategy for change: discourse analysis.

In this sense, the Foucauldian conceptualisation of 'discourse' challenges the concept of 'paradigm'. Deconstruction of the text reveals the politics inherent in both theory and methodology. The nature of the inquiry becomes the focus of inquiry. It is a strategy which transgresses the limitations of Marxist practice, where it is assumed that 'language bears a fixed and definite relationship with reality . . . language is regarded as a mere tool for communication' (Rojek et al. 1988: 118).

Foucault's discourse analysis reveals the objective construction of the person for the purpose of subjugation through 'dividing practices', including scientific classification. The range of social control has been extended since the seventeenth century through normalising knowledge systems which produce ascribed personal and social identities—such identities determining levels of social power and attracting disciplinary processes: violence, incarceration, poverty and so forth. However, Foucault is not limiting his approach to revealing symbols or signifying structures:

> Here I believe one's point of reference should not be to the great model of language (langue) and signs, but to that of war and battle. The history which bears and determines us has the form of a war rather than that of language: relations of power, not relations of meaning. (cited in Gordon 1980: 114)

As social workers, we needed to consider how our own practice might be divisive and how we could make it less so. Discourse analysis could unlock the power/knowledge nexus through an examination of the organisation of social institutions—specifically the production of heterogeneous textual positions which construct the basis of social relationships. The professional institution of social work can be included in these organisations.

FOUCAULT'S MAJOR CONTRIBUTION IS DISCOURSE ANALYSIS?

Discursive practices establish power relations. Power is produced historically through knowledge systems. Thus Foucault determines the historical construction of madness, sexuality and the prison—inquiring into the formulation of truths and the subsequent disciplining of people. He calls this a *genealogical* inquiry (Foucault 1979: 23).

It is a subjective process with objective outcomes. This disciplining process necessarily recruits people into maintaining their own subjugation—in actively participating in operations which shape their lives according to norms, even though those operations appear to be against their interests. For Foucault, power is productive. It subjects persons to normalising truths which shape their lives and relationships. It produces realities. As Billington (1991: 42) comments:

> concepts of normality apply to all sorts of ideas we have about ourselves and for which we set standards: 'a healthy body', 'a stable personality', 'sanity', 'a normal family', 'a proper man and woman' and so on. Moreover they institute new ways of exercising power through disciplinary mechanisms . . . psychological in character . . . through school rooms, welfare offices, hospitals, mental institutions, prisons, families and workplaces, through the cultural practices of welfare workers and others.

For Foucault, then, knowledge is power and subject positions are constructed through discourse. 'The individual which power has constituted is at the same time its vehicle' (Foucault in Gordon 1980: 98). Foucault thus offers an adequate account of people's toleration of, and participation in, oppressive power structures. This is often missing from other social theoretical analyses—liberal to radical.

WHAT IS FREIRE'S CONTRIBUTION?

The educational strategy of Freire provides the methodological framework for the teaching of interpersonal communication skills. Whilst there are differences between Foucault and Freire—for example, understandings of ideology—both involve transgressing the boundaries of positivism and both have inspired a tradition of writers from philosophy, psychology and education—and at last social work—who challenge the restraints imposed by science and humanism.

Foucault and Freire would concur on the notion of power and its social construction. They would also agree that poststructural ideas are a bridge between theory and practice, between a theory of social oppression and the practice of subjective change. Where Foucault uses discourse, Freire uses dialogue: the former is an analysis, the latter is an exchange to promote change. However, they both involve critical questioning. Freire uses the educational dialogical process to explore another person's subjective view 'communicating with each other not as objects being used by anyone . . . but in equality' (cited in Shor 1987: 223). Foucault uses discourse analysis to unsilence the process of 'use' and thus allow the construction of alternative social worlds.

The philosophy of Foucault complements the practice of

Freire. Freire has developed the critical dialogical techniques which can engage people in discovering the process suggested by Foucault. Freire is thus an educational bridge between Foucault and social work practice. Both integrate knowledge and power through the practice of criticism.

SO CRITICAL QUESTIONING IS INTRINSIC TO DISCOURSE ANALYSIS?

For Freire, critical education is part of the process of social change and this process is subjective and political: it is concerned with identifying who has power over whom and how it is maintained—with disclosing hegemony.

Without critical questioning, people continue to hold cultural meanings about the way their lives ought to be, even when their situations are oppressive. They may say: 'I'm not alright because I'm not like that', or 'I'm mad because the rest of the world act although they are not mad'. People tolerate these ideas, accepting what is called *doxa* in discourse analysis. This is:

> the prevailing view of things, which very often prevails to the extent that people are unaware that it is only one of several possible alternative views. (Sturrock 1979: 143)

For Freire, liberation from such a construction involves critically questioning the ideas which inform such an understanding—or model. He says:

> Intellectuals need ideas in order to understand the world but if these ideas become models . . . if they are not applied creatively . . . we run the risk of regarding them as reality . . . so concrete reality has to be made to fit in with our ideas and not the other way round. (Freire and Faundez 1990: 29)

For Foucault, the production of 'models' or 'truths' is discovered through a genealogical process:

> One has to dispense with the constituent subject, to get rid of the subject itself, that's to say, to arrive at an analysis which can account for the constitution of the subject within a historical framework. And this is what I would call genealogy, that is a form of history which can account for the constitution of knowledges, discourses, domains of objects, etc. (cited in Gordon 1980: 117)

Foucault's work critically targets the many forms of institutional technologies (for example, the Gulag, monarchy and prisons) through which disciplinary power systems are established.

Our experience was that social workers develop and use uncritical interpersonal communication models. In doing so, they are both discipliners and disciplined, conducting the interpersonal communication intervention process through a myriad of linguistic constructions including 'contracting', 'deprofessionalisation', 'help', 'support', 'problem solving', listening and empathy. This could well construct the subject of their own investigation, participating in the continual renewal of oppressive power and discrimination.

A formative text for us, which analysed this productive process in relation to education, was Walkerdine (1984). She examines a number of texts, including nursery record cards and teacher training content, within the context of conventional developmental psychology, medicalisation and normalisation. Walkerdine demonstrates that it is not that there is a 'pre-existent real object' (1984: 188)—in this case the developing child—which developmental psychology has 'distorted'. Rather, this is a decentred subject and it is:

> developmental psychology itself which produces the particular form of naturalised capacities as its object. The practices of production can, therefore, be understood as the production of subject-positions themselves. (1984: 164)

It is through such processes that educational powerlessness and its many material forms may be constructed. Those processes do not have within them the means of producing alternative ideas about the social world and consequent subject-positions. However, linguistically grounded social work (see Rojek et al. 1988) sees interpersonal communication become a primary focus for the process of critical questioning and social change. Here's Freire again:

> In communicating among ourselves, in the process of knowing the reality which we transform, we communicate and know socially even though the process of communicating, knowing, changing, has an individual dimension . . . Knowing is a social event with nevertheless an individual dimension. (Freire and Shor 1987: 99)

WHAT ARE THE MAJOR THEORETICAL DIFFERENCES BETWEEN THIS POSTSTRUCTURAL APPROACH AND THE HUMANIST APPROACH?

It is important to distinguish theoretically between different approaches to interpersonal communication. From the theoretical difference flows distinctive practice. For convenience, examine Table 11.1, which categorises difference while not implying exclusivity.

Table 11.1   Features of humanist and poststructural interpersonal communication approaches

Humanist	Poststructural
Linear	Lateral
Developmental	Genealogical
Centred subject	Decentred subject
Individual	Cultural
Therapeutic	Educational
Reformative	Diverse
Disciplining	Emancipatory
Normative	Critical
Causal	Archaeological
Reduction	Deconstruction
Self-actualise	Re-author

Humanist interpersonal communication practice is generally about exploring an individual problem, finding the psychosocial cause and identifying a solution which enables the client to operate more effectively and eventually achieve self-actualisation. It is therefore linear in its historical construction, developmental in conception and therapeutic and reformative in intent. Genealogically, this discursive position has its roots both in the secular confession and the cathartic psychoanalytical talking cure of Freud. This is the common discursive base to the various forms of casework, problem-solving and other strategies engaged by the social worker and mediated through the interpersonal communication process in the interview.

Prevailing humanist approaches are based on the notion of a self-contained unified subject. The intervention strategy utilised sees language as a reflection of the rational unified world to which we all belong. The goal is to find a way for the individual to 'self-actualise' within this given reality. This applies not only to Gerard Egan (982) or Bolton (1987), but also to radical structuralist (as distinct from poststructuralist) feminist and Marxist approaches which often seek to liberate people from a 'false consciousness'. Communication skills including listening, empathy, following and so on are seen as technical devices which enable a shared understanding of their purpose and impact. For this to occur, it is assumed that both the worker and the skills used are largely objective, neutral and facilitative.

A poststructural approach reconstructs the 'individual' as a 'vehicle and site' of cultural meaning. Language is the means of our subjectivity; it constructs multiple cultural meanings (including the very notion of one 'reality'). Subjectivity is at the same time constructed and producing meanings itself, primarily through discourses. This is the genealogy of Foucauldian philosophy applied to social work's interpersonal methodology.

A poststructural approach is therefore a decentred and discursive approach to theory and practice where history moves from a causal, binarist and linear past and present to a lateral archaeological critique of ideas and practices. The poststructural process deconstructs the genealogy of meaning, the process of subjectification, through a discourse analysis generating an archaeology of knowledge. Behaviours and their meanings are externalised, action is purposive rather than reactive and, as we shall see, technical interpersonal communication skills themselves are subject to this 'gaze'.

HOW DO YOU PRACTISE SKILLS WHICH DERIVE FROM THIS THEORY?

There are several practitioners persuaded by postmodernist ideas and critiques of humanist practice who influenced our work and which we have incorporated. These are the strengths perspective and restraints theory of Jenkins (1989), the narrative therapy of White (1991), the critical questioning approaches of Cooper (1994), Rossiter (1993), McGregor (1990) and Winslade et al. (1995) and the solution-focused work of Saleebey (1992) and Berg (1991).

White's methodology (see White 1986, 1988/89, 1991), including narrative therapy, involves externalising social/behavioural difficulties. White makes extensive use of Foucault's notion of the decentred subject, in removing relatively fixed qualities conventionally ascribed to persons and relationships. Indeed, this is perceived as the problem itself. The person's own story (narrative) determines the events they notice and the meaning they give to those events, rather than being seen as a reflection of their experience. White uses the notion of 'negative explanation' to question why things are not some other way. He asks what has prevented events from taking a different course, and what else is in the story which would allow a different conceptualisation of and response to the difficulties.

Alan Jenkins (1989) further translates socio-structural ideas into restraints and offers a practice of social change based on educational principles. Jenkins moves away from the historical reductionism of therapy and problem-solving. Beliefs are examined as barriers to alternative actions. The possibility of exploring alternative constructions of circumstances, rather than focusing on a presenting problem, is developed through a process of alternative (critical) questions.

McGregor's influential work in the area of domestic violence (see, for example, her 1990 critique of therapy), uses the ideas of Freire and Foucault and has been seminal in our work. McGregor has developed an interpersonal communication model taught to domestic violence workers, based on the principles discussed here, which again explicitly challenges traditional therapeutic models with their notions of internalised problems—a discourse in itself oppressive for women.

Rossiter (1993) and Winslade et al. (1995) have produced extensive material critically analysing the political context of interpersonal communication skills and making extensive use of Freirean critical questioning as a vehicle for exposing the political nature of beliefs and their impact on action

Dennis Saleebey (1992) has developed a strengths perspective in social work which again moves away from the 'problem-solving' approach. He connects both Freire and Foucault in identifying the need for this:

> Paulo Freire has maintained for many years that the views and expectations of oppressors have an uncanny and implacable impact on the oppressed, so that oppressed individuals and groups come to live and rationalise these tainted designations, subjugating their own knowledge and understanding to those of the oppressors. (1992: 4).

In Saleebey's work, alternative conditions are constructed between worker and interviewee which make it possible to work in an empowering way by developing potential rather than the magnifying of limitations produced by concentrating on deficits and pathologising them. This is not a simplistic version of thinking positively. The focus here is on engaging the person in a cognitive process informed by distinguishing what they can do and have done, in order to survive, change, control, contain their behaviour/circumstances. The process then establishes how to build on these strengths with action informed by different ideas.

Other writers, including Ann Weick (1992) and Insoo Kim Berg (1991), are also part of this transformation of practice. They provide a cogent critique of social work's domination by scientific 'received ideas' (Rojek et al. 1988)—specifically, a binarist, Cartesian, rational, objective, deficit interpretation of the social world. They offer strat-

Table 11.2 Practice strategies of humanist and poststructural interpersonal communication approaches

Humanist	Poststructural
Empathic responding	Critical questioning
Problem solving	Discourse analysis
Problem/deficit	Solution/strength
Affective	Cognitive
Pathology	Political culture
Participation	Restraint
Internalisation	Externalisation
Demonstrative language	Narrative language

egies which challenge social work's problem-saturated view of the world and they pose alternative reconceptualisations of cognitive, action-oriented, solution-focused methodologies which work with people's strengths and their ability to act on their worlds.

Utilising the work of Jenkins, White, McGregor and others mentioned here, students become concerned with the difference from the humanist problem-solving processes previously taken as absolute.

WHAT DID YOU ACTUALLY TEACH STUDENTS TO DO?

For us, discourse analysis constituted emancipatory practice within the interpersonal communication context. In short, such linguistic analysis discloses ideas, beliefs, norms, behaviours which produce normalisations—in effect, expressions of and [re]productions of prevailing power structures around race, class, gender, poverty, sexuality and so on. As social workers, we can collude with this or attempt ways to shift such discourses and their outcomes for individuals.

Skills in the interpersonal communication process are inquiries into knowledge and, as such, have a position in relation to the production of meanings and power with which social workers are concerned. Theories are vehicles of a discursive position: what is done/not done is a product of particular ideas/knowledge which exclude other knowledge. Skills are the instruments of that practice. Behaviours including language are expressions of these.

Previously, theory and practice had often been separated. Skills were learnt and practised within the parameters of an 'absolute' communication model—for example, Gerard Egan's 'Skills for Effective Helping' (Egan 1982). Now the discursive theory of informing and being informed by skills becomes identified: 'the notion of multiple realities of listening and being empathic now considered' (Levett 1997: 17). In this way, the popularly constructed binarism of theory and practice is deconstructed.

Let us take 'empathy' as an example. The interpersonal communication skills teacher has long used this skill. A popular understanding of empathy is that it enables the student/worker to understand another as if they were them and communicate this to them. However, if empathy is confined to a humanist discourse, it is mostly used with little revelation of its own political impact and production of particular knowledge/power social constructions. This is because its meaning is restricted to mirroring, a restriction that itself defines and limits its purpose, while still having other undeclared meanings and purposes.

We built on the work of Jan Fook (1993), which distinguished empathy from social empathy. Her notion of 'social' empathy is a major shift in declaring multiple meanings and political contexts—in this case, structural—to a communication skill. In seeking to apply poststructural principles to this skill, we needed to further distinguish the political contexts of empathy so that a postmodernist political analysis—that is the knowledge and power that using the skill produces, and is produced by—was revealed.

For teaching purposes, it is useful to conceptualise the skill of empathy in the following categorisations, each with their corollary discursive resonances. Using this knowledge, it is then possible to unravel the political stance of different approaches to interpersonal communication skills, including the political context of the skills inherent to various approaches.

Poststructural empathy is therefore the practice of discourse analysis in the interpersonal context, produced through critical questioning.

Table 11.3 Types of empathic responses in interpersonal communication

Emotional empathy	The expression of another person's feelings in relation to personal situation
Social empathy	The revelation of the relationship between another's feelings and ideas (thinking) and their social context and its material impact
Structural empathy	The disclosure of another's situation in relation to socio-structural normalisation processes
Post-structural empathy	The clarification of the discourses through which another constructs their power positions, meanings and behaviours in relation to normalisation processes

CAN YOU OFFER AN EXAMPLE OF THIS?

We will use a case study example. B is now separated from her partner following a violent, disruptive relationship. They have four children aged from five years down, who are all in care and have suffered emotional and physical abuse, although it is not clear whether the perpetrator is B or her former partner. All four male children were between six and eight weeks premature and this is consistent with abuse of alcohol and prescription drugs. There is no information which says that B hails from a violent family background. At this time, both parents are at war over access to the children. One child has been returned to the mother's care. The mother has moved into a shelter and is undergoing counselling from a feminist group.

The following demonstrates contrasting questions which can produce different analytical discourses for the client. They are categorised here within the distinct empathic types.

Emotional

'Can you tell me what happened and how you feel about this?'
'How has the problem got worse?'
'Can we explore your feelings about your relationship, separation from the children and how you can put your life back together for their return?'

Social

'Let's talk about what supports are available to you—for example, family, community, friends.'
'Can you describe your relationship with these supports and how you feel about them?'
'What work is available to you and what is your opinion about working?'
'How can you manage financially on your own?'
'How do you think that alcohol and drugs are damaging for you?'
'What can you do about this damage . . . what support systems are there?'

Structural

'What kind of control have men had over your life?'
'Can you tell me what rights you believe you have as a mother, wife and individual?'
'Can we explore how this violence started?'

'What sort of control do you believe social security and the welfare have over you?'

'What resources do you need to get your children back?'

Poststructural

'Tell me what you think the role of mother and partner should be.'

'Where do these expectations come from?' 'How do you differ from these?'

'If we accept that men have it better, nevertheless, what control do you have in your situation?'

'How do you think this kind of control could keep you in this situation?'

'How can you think in a different way about your children and partner so that your control is not damaging for you and others?'

'How do you exercise power and violence in your life?'

'What do you do that you think maintains the violence in your relationship with your children and others?'

'We have talked about your rights. We can agree that they include safety, love, adequate finances. Can you tell me what responsibilities you think you have towards others with regard to these?'

The objective with questioning using a poststructural approach is to help the interviewee elucidate what it is about their own ideas and behaviours which enables them to participate in a situation that is destructive for them. In this sense, they are not only 'surviving', but themselves re/producing a political structure which both disciplines them and punishes; which constructs their own prison.

This shift in knowledge offers the production of a different *form* of power. This does not deny the material personal and political suffering of this client, nor the role played by others in the way power has been produced between them. Indeed, this form of interpersonal questioning needs to occur with all in the social work system, not only with 'the client'.

In practice, each form of questioning has importance and a poststructural approach *builds on to*—rather than operating *instead of*—a structural one. In this way, it effects change in normalisation processes such as gender, class and race—first at the subjective level and then in the material world. As Weedon (1987: 19) comments:

> I would argue the appropriateness of poststructuralism to feminist concerns, not as the answer to *all* feminist questions but as a way

of conceptualising the relationship between language, social institutions and individual consciousness which focuses on how power is exercised and the possibilities of change.

HOW DID YOU STRUCTURE THE TEACHING?

We taught interpersonal communication skills across two modules. In the first module, students learnt basic skills such as listening, following and responding. At the same time, we began to engage students in critically analysing the theoretical basis of various writers, including psychoanalytic theorists as well as Barber (1991), Fook (1993), Bolton (1987), Egan (1982) and Freire (1987) using the Burrell and Morgan (1979) paradigms. Although this formulation can be dismissed as a structuralist device, as a construct it can also be used in a poststructuralist way by enabling a rudimentary 'discourse analysis' of these communication theories and practices. The second module taught students the specifics of postmodern theory and practice discussed in this chapter.

Basic principles of the work of the aforementioned writers, including Foucault, Freire and the interpersonal communication skills proponents White, Jenkins, MacGregor, Weick, Rossiter, Berg and Saleebey, were presented and their contributions analysed in relation to supporting individual and social change.

Students were required to produce a comparative analysis of different interpersonal communication approaches employed within different services in the industry by researching and reporting on the different methodologies used in agencies and their relationship to the philosophy of the agency. Students were taught to conduct a range of structured interviews integrating the following skills:

- Establish rapport and contact appropriately.
- Validate concerns and feelings.
- Follow the client's narrative/story.
- Work with the present situation.
- Support the client to:
  - investigate strengths and restraints;
  - explore options;
  - make decisions.
- Integrate critical questioning by
  - locating the structural ideas and behaviours in the narrative;
  - connecting this knowledge/power nexus to individual and structural oppression.

- Demonstrate emotional/social/(post)structural empathy.
- Explore alternative discourses with the interviewee.

Students were taught critical reflection through analysis of their use of self. This involved evaluation of their values and use of power and authority within the interpersonal communication context of the total learning environment and was conducted by both student and teacher in structured exercises and classroom interactions. Learners were required to engage in critical reflection of their learning by distinguishing their learning constraints, formulating strategies to address those constraints and implementing those strategies. The teacher was required to provide the feedback to assist with this. Assessment was based on the student being able to successfully demonstrate the above skills and complete the required tasks.

ARE THERE ANY SPECIFIC TEACHING SKILLS AND STRATEGIES USED WITH THIS APPROACH?

While there are significant differences (e.g. assessment) the teacher/student relationship often reflects the worker/client context. Both approaches are educational and discursive rather than therapeutic. We sought to reproduce this within the learning environment.

Teaching needs to avoid the humanist pitfalls outlined above, such as the black hole of historical causation and problem-solving. Additionally, students are required to deconstruct their own narratives through everyday language concerning 'private troubles and public issues'. This is often confronting, and therefore requires a highly structured learning environment with clearly identified assessment criteria, demonstration of differences between theoretical approaches, explicitly targeted exercises offered by the teacher and examples of current workplace practices where postmodern approaches are used.

Formative assessment is essential. We accomplished this with an ongoing video record of each student's practice attempts across the module as well as continuous written and verbal feedback. Reflective journalling, learning contracts and behaviourally measured feedback are further examples of teaching strategies used.

CONCLUSION

In this chapter, we invited our anonymous interlocutor to ask questions which would allow us to deconstruct the dominant humanist discursive position that had informed our teaching and practice of interpersonal communication skills. This brief genealogy disclosed how certain concepts have been constructed to produce an oppressive, rather than liberating, social work practice. We then argued that an alternative discourse and practice are possible, which coherently address the primary concern of our profession: personal and social change.

We have developed an approach which integrates poststructural Foucauldian discourse analysis and Freirean educational practice. This produces a distinctly postmodern and decentred dimension to social work, which retains the importance of individual material conditions in its interpersonal context, while seeking genuine radical change in society.

REFERENCES

Barber, J. (1991) *Beyond Casework*, Macmillan, Basingstoke

Berg, I.K. (1991) *Family Based Services: A Solution Focused Approach*, W.W. Norton, New York

Billington, R. (1991) *Culture and Society: A Sociology for Culture*, Macmillan Education, London

Bolton, R. (1987) *People Skills,* Simon & Schuster, Brookvale

Burrell, G. and Morgan, G. (1979) *Sociological Paradigms and Organisational Analysis*, Heinemann, London

Calinescu, M. (1987) *Five Faces of Modernity*, Duke University Press, Durham

Cooper, L. (1994) 'Critical Story Telling in Social Work Practice', *Australian Journal of Adult and Community Education*, vol. 34, no. 2, pp. 131–40

Egan, G. (1982) *The Skilled Helper*, Brooks & Cole, Monterey

Fischer, M.M.J. and Marcuse, G.E. (1986) *Anthropology as Cultural Critique: An Experimental Moment in the Human Sciences*, University of Chicago Press, Chicago

Fook, J. (1993) *Radical Casework: A Theory of Practice*, Allen & Unwin, Sydney

——(ed.) (1996) *The Reflective Researcher: Social Workers' Theories of Practice*, Allen & Unwin, Sydney

Foucault, M. (1979) *Discipline and Punish*, Penguin, Harmondsworth

Freire, P. and Shor, I. (1987) *A Pedagogy for Liberation: Dialogues on Transforming Education*, Macmillan, Cambridge

Freire, P. and Faundez, A. (1990) *Learning to Question: A Pedagogy of Liberation*, WCC Publications, Geneva

Gordon, C. (1980) *Power/Knowledge: Selected Interviews and Other Writings 1972–1977: Michel Foucault*, Harvester, Brighton

Horton, M. and Freire, P. (1990) *We Make the Road by Walking: Conver-*

sations on Education and Social Change, Temple University Press, Philadelphia

Jenkins, A. (1989) *Invitations to Responsibility*, Dulwich Centre Publications, Adelaide

Levett, P. (1997) The Interface Between Poststructuralism and Competency Based Training, with Particular Reference to the Implications for Assessment in an Environment of Flexible Delivery, unpublished MEd thesis, University of Tasmania, Hobart

McGregor, H. (1990) 'Conceptualising Male Violence Against Female Partners: Political Implications of Therapeutic Responses', *Australia and New Zealand Journal of Family Therapy*, vol. 11, no. 2, pp. 65–70

Lonsdale, M. (1991) Postmodernism and the Study of History, unpublished MEd thesis, La Trobe University, Melbourne

Peters, M. (ed.) (1995) *Education and the Postmodern Condition*, Bergin and Garvey, Westwood

Rabinow, P. (ed.) (1984) *The Foucault Reader*, Penguin, Harmondsworth

Rojek, C., Peacock, G. and Collins, S. (1988) *Social Work and Received Ideas*, Routledge, London

Rossiter, A. (1993) 'Teaching from a Critical Perspective: Towards Empowerment in Social Work Education', *Canadian Social Work Review*, vol. 10, no. 1, pp. 76–90

Saleebey, D. (1992) *The Strengths Perspective in Social Work Practice*, Longman, New York

Shor, I. (1987) *Freire for the Classroom*, Boynton/Cook Publishing, Heinemann, Portsmouth

Sturrock, J. (1979) (ed.) *Structuralism and Since*, Oxford University Press, Oxford

Walkerdine, V. (1984) 'Developmental Psychology and the Child Centred Pedagogy: The Insertion of Piaget into Early Education', J. Henriques, W. Holloway, C. Urwin, C. Venn and V. Walkerdine (eds), *Changing the Subject: Psychology, Social Regulation and Subjectivity*, Methuen, London

Weedon, C. (1987) *Feminist Practice and Poststructural Theory*, Blackwell, Oxford

Weick, A. (1992) 'Building a Strengths Perspective in Social Work' in D. Saleeby (ed.), *The Strengths Perspective in Social Work Practice*, Longman, White Plains

White, M. (1986) 'Negative Explanation, Restraint and Double Description: A Template for Family Therapy', *Family Process*, no. 25, p. 2

——(1988/89) 'The Externalising of the Problem and the Reauthoring of Lives and Relationships', *Dulwich Centre Newsletter*, Summer, Adelaide, pp. 3–21

——(1991) 'Deconstruction and Therapy', *Dulwich Centre Newsletter*, no. 3, Adelaide, pp. 21–40

Winslade, J., Drewery, W. and Monk, G. (1995) Sharpening the Critical Edge: A Social Constructionist Approach in Counsellor Education, unpublished, University of Waikato, Hamilton

12 Competing paradigms in mental health practice and education
Lister Bainbridge

Social sciences cannot eschew their inferior status until they reject the epistemology which defines them as inferior (Hekman 1990: 8)

INTRODUCTION

The impetus for this chapter arose from the reworking of the Bachelor of Social Work (BSW) and the Bachelor of Community Welfare (BCW) degrees at James Cook University in Queensland which has taken place over the last four years. A curriculum review group was appointed to produce revised programs for both degrees.

Our department (now a School of Social Work and Community Welfare) was until recently a part of the School of Behavioural Sciences, which over the years had projected a strong positivist psychology component into social welfare studies, along with an emphasis on quantitative research methods. The new curriculum has attempted to redress this imbalance by providing a rounded, holistic curriculum with an increased emphasis on qualitative inquiry.

An important example of this imbalance was the inclusion of a psychopathology subject as a compulsory unit for final year BSW students. The content and teaching of this subject were designed much more to meet the needs of the Australian Psychological Society than to prepare social work students for mental health practice. Lecture material focused almost entirely around an abnormal psychology framework, with strong emphasis placed on studying the *DSMIV* (*Diagnostic and Statistical Manual*, 4th edition, American Psychiatric Association, 1994) and, although there was a critique of this diagnostic approach, there still seemed to be an uncritical acceptance of the biomedical model.

For students, this subject reinforced perceptions already held,

179

and perhaps internalised, that the real expertise in mental health
lay somewhere else—in the province of psychiatry and the neuro-
sciences. This in turn made it more difficult for them to assimilate
mental health work into their own practice, let alone to make it
an integral part of a personal philosophy of practice.

This incompatibility of contexts is the main theme of this
chapter, which looks at how a more relevant recontextualisation
can be provided which fits better into the socio-political framework of social welfare practice. The chapter begins with a look
at some postmodernist concepts relevant to this theme. Second,
the implications of these ideas for the arena of sanity and madness
are discussed. From here, some areas of research and practice
relevant to social work and mental health are briefly explored.
The chapter finishes with a discussion of the application of these
ideas in relation to social work and the mental health curriculum.

THE POSTMODERN CONTEXT

The dark Satanic mills of William Blake both reflected and signalled the onset of industrialism and modernity. Modernism was
concerned with the grand narratives and the search for universal
theories and truths heralded by the Enlightenment. Big was good,
mainstream came to become automatically right. Western industrial democracies came to see themselves as some sort of normative
yardstick. This yardstick was then used to examine and interpret
other, less 'developed', societies. However, 'today, the view is
spreading that modernity itself, far from being a normative yardstick is a historical stage to be overcome on the way to a
post-modern or post-industrial society' (Benhabib 1992: 68).

The self-satisfied and arrogant notion of the big theory has
apparently come unstuck because of its selective epistemological
base. Postmodernists contrast, for example, the grand narratives
of the Enlightenment with the 'petit recits' of women, children,
fools and primitives. These 'small stories' or 'web of stories' were
excluded from the grandiose version of the modern Western
tradition (Sarup 1993). As Seyla Benhabib comments (1992: 14):

> If there is one commitment which unites postmodernists from
> Foucault to Derrida to Lyotard, it is the critique of Western
> rationality as seen from the perspective of the margins, from the
> standpoint of what and whom it excludes, suppresses,
> deligitimizes, renders mad, imbecilic or childish.

In other words, postmodernists challenge the binary system of
oppositions with its corollary of domination and subordination.

This binary system and its associated discursive practices can lead to socially constructed distinctions between mental health and mental disorder, normal and criminal behaviour, and madness and civilisation. These distinctions always imply the existence of 'the other' as a reference point. The problem here is that 'the other' is constructed through constructions of self. So, for example, the orientalism of Edward Said (1995) is a Western construct of 'the other' as primitive and inferior. Anthropologists appropriate the stories of 'the other'. Is this to understand and to explain differences, or to maintain and amplify them? This subordination, of course, applies to all people on the margins, including women, children, fools and primitives.

The questions that strike me as important here are:

- Can any identity be constructed without reference to difference?
- Is the logic of binary oppositions always a logic of subordination and domination?

SANITY AND MADNESS: POWER AND KNOWLEDGE

Is there a universal entity called sanity in opposition to another universally recognisable entity called madness? Everyone has their own idea about this, and their own ontology. But each of us is limited to what we are and know, and where we have come from. Into whatever culture we are born, we are socialised to absorb and internalise the way in which our culture is ordered and manifested (Bradley 1989). Part of this includes ontologies of sanity and madness.

We see, over periods of history, a range of ontologies—sometimes recurring. For example, the notion of madness as divine election, divine intervention or supernatural possession was prevalent in pre-Classical Greece and then in pre-Renaissance Europe. Other periods have seen madness as folly, sin and moral degeneracy. And, of course, the word lunacy derives from an astrophysical ontology! The point here is that not all of these ontologies were in the form of a binary opposition intended to subordinate and devalue.

Ideas such as these never exist in a vacuum and their variation over time may be linked to particular political and material interests of the period and the prevailing culture (Warner 1994; Thomas 1997). Whatever the case, ideas in their structural manifestations can exert enormous power over human lives (Banton et al. 1985).

The rise of industrialism in the nineteenth century was accompanied by a rapid increase in institutional structures, the function of which was to maintain and protect power and order in the emerging capitalist society. This was the period of the great incarcerations which saw increased separatism: the movement of mad people into asylums, conscripts into barracks, the criminally deviant into prisons and, of course, children into schools. These processes and structures were much more discreet than the previous public displays of criminals and lunatics. New areas of professional expertise began to develop and the acquired knowledge became an instrument for the development and maintenance of power. For Foucault (1967), forms of knowledge such as psychiatry and criminology are directly related to the exercise of power. There is a spiral of power and knowledge in which political economy directs the development of knowledge while at the same time professional knowledge may or may not become the producer of positive change. This power itself creates new objects of knowledge and accumulates new bodies of information which are not necessarily in the public interest (Cohen 1985). 'The conceiving of power as repression, constraint or prohibition is inadequate (for Foucault): power produces reality, it produces domains of objects and rituals of truth' (Sarup 1993: 74).

The way this happens is not through a straightforward, top-down approach 'where those in authority exert various forms of coercive restraint upon the mass of more or less compliant subjects' (Sarup 1993: 74). Rather, the control of knowledge is secured by persuading us to internalise the norms and values that prevail within the dominant social order and which then become paradigmatic. I shall refer to this internalisation process later in relation to the mental health curriculum.

I would now like to look at these ideas in relation to the concepts of mental health and mental illness—in particular, how in this arena in modern society, power has come to direct knowledge rather than the reverse. The idea of power directing knowledge has many manifestations in this arena and I would like to explore a few examples which are relevant both to the postmodernist debate regarding binary oppositions and to a mental health education curriculum.

PSYCHOPHARMACOLOGICAL RESEARCH

Of all the money given over to mental health research, by far the greatest amount is directed to psychopharmacology in the search for biological correlates (or causes) of mental disorder and even better symptom-relieving pills. As Kleinman (1988: 73) comments, 'biology has cachet with psychiatrists; anthropology and sociology do not'. I like the use of the word 'cachet' here: according to *Chambers' Dictionary*, it means both 'something showing or conferring prestige' and 'a capsule containing a medicine'.

The dilemma is that there is considerable evidence pointing to the social origins of depression (see, for example, Brown and Harris 1978), and no clear-cut findings pointing to biological causes. Yet there is a systematic resistance to dealing with social sources of depression and other psychiatric conditions. There is thus a clear bias in psychiatry in the very way knowledge is created, so that social causes and social remedies are minimised and even denied. Further, this bias is given support from a range of sectors in society. The discovery of the latest magic pill is greeted with enthusiasm by the media. In the process, the public is led to believe that biology has the answers to emotional problems. Families of the mentally ill may find support from biological causes which suggest emotional disturbance is just another illness; this may reduce the burden of guilt. In the process, allied professionals—including social workers—may derive enhanced career prospects through this empire.

It does not seem to matter, as Cohen (1985) points out, that huge amounts of money are spent on both criminological and psychiatric research, with very few definitive results. Drug companies sponsor hundreds of research papers each year to show that trademarked products are superior to others. The conclusion of most papers is that there are no medically significant differences. No matter: the point has been made. Mental health education needs to address these themes.

ETHNOPSYCHIATRY RESEARCH

In the textbooks of psychiatry, there seems to be a general implicit agreement that mental illness is prevalent in all cultures. It is presented almost as common knowledge, paradigmatic, something we can take as a given, and rarely supported by convincing evidence. In turn, this reinforces the grand narrative of sanity and madness as universal truth. It also supports the essentialist idea that human beings are born with some intact personality, a psychic structure which renders some people prone to mental illness and others not. Madness is a long-term static state rather than a complex dynamic process. All of this, of course, promotes the biogenic ontology, and the assumed worldwide prevalence of mental illness is used in support. The grand narrative remains intact.

Certainly, there is evidence which points in this direction. The question concerns the extent to which it stands up to analysis (see, for example, Marshall 1988). Different cultures have different ways of responding to life's stresses at individual and social levels, which can only be interpreted in relation to the complexities of a specific culture, its signs and symbols. Those of us who dispute the binary categories of sanity and madness have a problem with the image of an ethnopsychiatric researcher, armed with the *DSMIV*, travelling to far-away societies. It may be that the researcher cannot speak the language of that society, let alone know much about the complexities of its culture. Yet, nonetheless, behaviour is observed which matches the symptoms of schizophrenia as defined by the *DSMIV*. Mere observations of 'the other', with or without an understanding of the context, support the grand theory. An added problem is that most of these studies not only export, use and incorporate the biogenic ontology of Western culture as a yardstick, but virtually always do so after the culture being studied has fallen victim to acculturation processes.

Other researchers argue differently (see, for example, Devereux 1987; Kleinman 1988; Warner 1994). Warner, for example, produces evidence to show that the occurrence and course of schizophrenia are strongly conditioned by the political economy. Unemployment and economic depression in the West and the development of capitalist modes of wage-labour in non-Western societies appear to lead to greater numbers of people showing symptoms of schizophrenia, and fewer of them improving. Prevalence is lower where wage labour has not developed. He supports this in making a correlation between the increase in wage labour during industrialism and the rise in the occurrence of schizophrenia in the industrialised West. In gender terms, he notes a connection between the age of onset of schizophrenia and the age at which women and men enter the labour market. Curiously, there seems to be here, in relation to schizophrenia, the idea of a cultural double bind somewhat analogous to that of the family double bind put forward by Bateson (1973) and others.

These ideas are supported by the French ethnopsychiatrist George Devereux (1987), who argues that, in many pre-colonisation societies, schizophrenia, as we define it, did not exist. He based his evidence on work done with societies prior to, or at the point of, invasive acculturation. He predicts, however, that following this invasion, schizophrenia will become a common functional disorder because of the dramatic changes in the ecological, social and interpretive elements of the culture. Closer to home, the work by Morice (1978) with the Pintupe people in central Australia showed that they had a sophisticated vocabulary describing emotional states including anger, fear, anxiety, depression and shame, but not psychotic states. A similar notion was alluded to in the report of the House of Representatives Standing Committee on Aboriginal Affairs in 1979 (HRSCAA: 131):

> Professor Cawte gave the committee evidence which suggested that mental illnesses were experienced in Aboriginal communities before contact with whites but that these were essentially different from those presently predominant.

Work undertaken by Erich Fromm (1973) looked at the studies carried out on some 30 different societies by anthropologists. Fromm was able to describe these societies in three categories: life-affirmative societies; non-destructive, aggressive societies; and destructive societies. The differences here may relate to the differences Warner (1994) noted in pre- and post-industrialised societies and may also relate to ideas expressed earlier in the century by Roheim (1930) regarding what he called the therapeutically orientated society. As an aside, one intriguing idea emerging from writers such as Devereux (1987) is the level of involuntariness of psychotic states, and whether some societies practised ritualistic enactment of psychotic states as a preventive, prophylactic process. While perhaps beyond the scope of this chapter, there are certainly insights here into the intricate relationship between culture and mental health and, in my view, mental health education needs to address these themes.

INSTITUTIONS, LABELLING, POWER AND KNOWLEDGE

The great incarcerations of the nineteenth century were projects of segregation, normalisation, control, discipline and surveillance. They also led to an obsession with classification: taxonomies of people, as well as butterflies and other creatures. Unfortunately, the great energies were used to create and classify abnormal behaviour rather than to eliminate it. This roller-coaster seems unstoppable. As Cohen (1985: 99) comments, 'it is difficult to see how modern social control systems can do anything but expand . . . Each stage creates the correctional clients it wants.' I would add that it also treats them in what Illich (1976) calls 'iatrogenic feedback loops'.

An example of this comes from a study by Mendel and Rapport (1969) into reasons for admissions into psychiatric institutions.

This study found no correlation between severity of symptoms and the decision regarding admission, even when the admitting professionals thought there was. The most significant indicator of admission was whether the person had been in a psychiatric hospital before. This is the iatrogenic feedback loop, similar to the concept of amplification of deviance (Scheff 1966) in labelling theory. Foucault (1967) takes this further: the institution has nothing to do with turning mad people into sane people, bad people into good people. Rather, there is another, darker side where institutional power amplifies deviance and thereby distorts perceived public knowledge. The institution is more than just a depository for its inmates. Those who reject the binary system of sanity and madness might argue that, in a continuum of emotional states, all of us have mad 'bits' and bad 'bits'. The institution then becomes a depository for these as well, leaving those of us 'outside' feeling saner and 'gooder'. The social construction of the 'other' has the follow-on effect of modifying the social construction of 'self'. Thus the institution affects how we see ourselves and amplifies the difference between 'us' and 'them', thus confirming the knowledge of the classifiers. The public then sees institutions as a source of relief and security, as well as centres of professional knowledge and power.

This acknowledgment is reflected in public spending where until recently in Western countries, an average of 90–95 per cent of public money was spent on the 5–10 per cent of the people in need in institutions, leaving 5–10 per cent of public money for the 90–95 per cent of people in need in the community. The state obviously is prepared to spend a lot of money on who decides who's mad and pays them very well (Caplan 1995).

It goes without saying that psychiatric units are generally in hospitals—or called hospitals—thereby reinforcing the biogenic ontology. Unfortunately, in any psychological sense, practices can often be anti-therapeutic and lack the rationality which many attribute to them. Rather, there is ritualistic pragmatism of the kind where the nurse wakes a patient to take a sleeping pill or where the nursing home residents are woken up before dawn to take a bath to fit in with the nursing rota. The salient features of good therapeutic group practice—democratisation, communalism, permissiveness and reality confrontation (Rapoport 1960)—become very difficult to operate, even with the best-intentioned staff. All of this, however, can be seductive to the paramedic professionals such as social workers, who far too easily can get caught up in what Cohen (1985) calls the master patterns. Mental health education needs to address these themes.

GENDER

> Normal men have killed about 100,000,000 other normal men in the last fifty years. (R.D. Laing)

Textbooks of psychiatry and abnormal psychology exhibit such a thundering silence on issues of gender and mental health that one has to question the reasons for this omission. Is the medicalisation of women's health too much a political hot potato for the experts to discuss? Or does it never dawn on them that the social construction of masculinity and feminity is just as much a part of the system of binary oppositions in industrial society as is that of sanity and madness? Do they see the grand narrative on sanity and madness as gender-neutral? Do they consider the DSMIV *not* to be a gender biased social construction? I think the answer to all these questions is in the affirmative.

Most of what little mainstream research on mental health and gender has been done is very recent. Earlier, Brown and Harris (1978) showed very clearly the effects of the subservient role of women in our society on mental health. Yet women continue to be bombarded with a startling array of highly addictive tranquillising drugs to help them to maintain their subservient role. By labelling their distress as a clinical problem rather than an understandable reaction to role stresses, psychiatry serves the interests of patriarchal capitalism.

It is only in recent years that connections have been made between other areas of domination and mental health—for example, the connection between child sexual abuse and anorexia, bulimia and prostitution (see, for example, Zerbe 1993). Not surprisingly, this work has come much more from feminist scholars than from mainstream mental health professionals. I am reminded here of that American study where the attributes of mentally healthy adults generally were perceived by clinical mental health workers to be much more closely akin to the attributes of mature adult males than to those of mature adult females (Broverman et al. 1970). Yet these apparently straightforward studies appear to have been studiously ignored.

In relation to mental health and gender, I have carried out an exercise with our social work students for the last few years. Students divide into about seven or eight different groups and adopt roles: conventional psychiatrist, psychiatric nurse, Mr and Mrs Average, psychiatric patient, social worker, therapeutic community worker/client, socialist feminist, radical feminist. I ask them to think about what mental health means in their respective roles and report back to the larger group with three or four ideas of what constitutes positive mental health from their perspective. What emerges is a refutation of the grand narrative from a gender perspective. From the perspective of the dominant paradigm, positive mental health is seen to be conformity to the gender, occupational and behavioural norms of our society. From other perspectives, positive mental health is seen to include the ability to throw off the gendered expectations of a patriarchal society. From these contrasting views of what exactly positive mental health is, students are able to reflect on where they stand and what this means in terms of emancipatory practice. This in turn raises questions for the class about concepts such as normalisation, as well as issues regarding planning for effective community care in the mental health arena.

The equal-and-the-same versus the equal-but-different debate is still going on. What I do know is that men have to assist women in the process of setting up support units which do not operate from the implicit assumption of binary oppositions—in conflict-resolution terms, those which operate from a win–win position (hard on the problem, soft on the people) rather than a win–lose position (soft on the problem, hard on the people). Feminist workers have already embarked on this process. Where are the men? Mental health education needs to address these themes.

THE DISABILITY LOBBY

My last example is to do with the conceptualisation of emotional problems as disability, rather than illness. There is no question that the human rights component in the disability lobby has helped to raise the status of disabled people as well as to raise the consciousness of social welfare workers in this domain. The study of disability is now approached by students with more commitment than before because of its link with advocacy and active social change. However, until recently, this commitment has been mainly confined to the areas of physical and intellectual disability, with comparatively little attention paid to psychiatric disability in this context.

This lack of response is apparent at different levels. For welfare workers, it may be that physical and intellectual disabilities are perceived to be more an integral part of 'their' domain, whereas psychiatric disability is in the province of others; this may have actually been reinforced in their own professional training. For psychiatrists and the drug industrialists, it would mean a massive epistemological shift away from their entrenched power bases, the institutions and the hospitals. For governments, it means a vote-losing challenge against the huge vested interests of multi-national companies and the medical associations, although other reasons such as cost (not correct) are given as excuses. For the public, it means confronting the possibility of all those projections into institutions coming back into the community to haunt us.

My concern here in relation to mental health education is that we need well-trained, strong and committed workers in community care who can help prevent the transportation of many of the pathogenic features of the institutions to the community, as seems already to be happening in the United States and elsewhere (Fuller Torrey 1997). I feel strongly that there is an important role here for social work, which may well be the profession best equipped for the task.

Deconstruction takes time, and perhaps reconstruction is a huge challenge given all these vested interests. Certainly community care has a lot going for it from a social justice, emancipatory perspective, but much stacked against it.

BACK TO POSTMODERNISM

The examples I've given here sound like a catalogue of tasks in the process of deconstruction. Can postmodernism offer anything more than cogent arguments for deconstruction? Does postmodernism have a politics? What can it offer in the way of reconstruction?

I think many of us have ambivalent feelings about postmodernism. Are we part of a baby boomer philosophy, blasé about all the privileges of modernism which we enjoy? Is postmodernism a critique without a politics or a future direction or a theory of action? Certainly it has made people stop and think. Certainly it has legitimised areas where many of us felt that we were the odd person out, had counter-establishment views or feelings of alienation or perceptions of heresy. As Seyla Benhabib (1992: 15) puts it: 'Postmodernism, in its infinitely sceptical and subversive attitude toward normative claims, institutional justice and political struggles is certainly refreshing. Yet, it is also debilitating.' Or as Antonio Gramsci (1977) put it as far back as the 1920s:

> The crisis consists precisely in the fact that the old is dying and the new cannot be born; in this interregnum a great variety of morbid symptoms appear . . . the death of the old ideologies takes the form of scepticism with regards to all theories and general formulae in and to a form of politics which is not simply realistic

in fact (this is always the case) but which is cynical in its immediate manifestation.

Does it flatter to deceive, to convey visions of hope without the formula for achieving it? Or will the dark Satanic mills haunt us for an eternity lasting a lot longer than an hour?

IMPLICATIONS FOR SOCIAL WORK AND THE MENTAL HEALTH CURRICULUM

What do these competing ontologies and values tell us in relation to mental health education and practice for social workers? Are they in terminal collision mode, or can they be accommodated?

Australia is one of a number of countries which, over the last few decades, has been reviewing its mental health policies in terms of the balance of institutional and community care, which previously saw the largest slice of the spending cake given over to institutional care for a relatively small minority of the people in need. Various kinds of policy papers have signalled the intention to transfer substantial amounts of funding towards community care to help redress this serious imbalance (see, for example, Human Rights and Equal Opportunities Commission 1993). For those of us in the field of social work, this should be good news. There should be opportunities here to develop and expand new, holistic models of mental health practice which are congruent with the social justice perspectives fundamental to our codes of ethics and values.

Unfortunately, it is not that simple, as the ideas offered in this chapter might suggest. Vested interests of power underlying competing ontologies of sanity and madness inevitably lead to practice problems in relation to professional demarcation and territory. These problems have now become compounded by the juggernaut of economic rationalism which wants, *inter alia*, to privatise everything, regardless of outcomes to people in need.

How can these complicating factors inform our practice as social workers? Let's try to summarise these values in collision. On the one hand, we have discontinuous models of sanity and madness. These fit comfortably with capitalism, because they promote the binary opposition of 'us and them', which serves to maintain a dominant–subordinate, win–lose set of relationships so important for capitalism. They fit well with the climate of rampant individualism. They promote nature over nurture and use selective, ideologically driven research to promote as paradigmatic that schizophrenia is inherited, genetic, a disease, and universally responsive to neuroleptic drugs. They see mental illness as a one-person event, which, allied with economic rationalism, encourages case management, case mix, institutional care, quality control and competency-based training. They really have no interest in looking at the relationships between health, mental health, social factors and the political economy, and at the extreme end see community mental health as a threat to professional identity and power.

On the other hand, we have continuous models of sanity and madness which suggest, rather, a continuum of mental health and disorder in all of us, and try to break down the dominant–subordinate set of relations of the expert-consumer. They eschew the binary opposition of 'us and them', and do not fit comfortably with capitalism and rampant individualism. They promote nurture and social factors above nature and the genetic disease model, and encourage research looking at social, gender, economic and political factors in individual distress. They have a healthy disrespect for vested global research dollars such as those of multinational drug companies. Finally, they wish to promote, develop and expand holistic models of mental health practice in ways which recognise the inherent self-worth of every individual and which involve consumers in self-help groups, research and policy planning.

Although this catalogue of contrasting paradigms is somewhat caricatured, it nonetheless constitutes, in my view, a useful framework of reference as a starting point in the curriculum for students of a final-year social work and mental health subject, where the primary aim is to help students to assimilate mental health work into their own personal philosophy of practice.

So, in developing the new subject 'Social Work and Mental Health', the first epistemological aim was to find ways of examining with the students our own assumptive world, the world which shapes our own individual ontology of sanity and madness. How and why have we come (as is nearly always the case) to internalise the dominant paradigm which sees madness and badness contained almost totally within the notion of individual pathology, and therefore requiring individual one-on-one 'treatment' from an expert somewhere else? The power of this is very strong and hard to throw off, I've found (Bainbridge 1985), in spite of students being well advanced on a social work degree.

Fortunately, the power of self-discovery is also very strong, and this process leads to enormous gains in how students approach the subject. The framework shifts from the remote to contemplating the inner and the outer, the personal and the political (Holmes 1992). I have found this ontological shift to be by far and away the most important educational hurdle and the excitement of discovery can be quite tangible.

The second objective is to survey the social, cultural, economic and political contexts of mental health practice. This is where the areas of anthropology, feminism, psychoanalysis and postmodernism are important. These are, not surprisingly, the very areas which powerful professional bodies such as the Royal College of Psychiatry in the United Kingdom view with suspicion (Thomas 1997). It is my view, however, that without at least some understanding of the contribution of these areas, the connections between economic rationalism, the political economy and mental health are not easy to clarify. This process also facilitates in students an awareness of how the power and knowledge spiral creates a systematic bias in the production of information which eventually becomes paradigmatic.

Third, and as a consequence of the above, students need to be aware of, and tolerant towards, both the knowledge bases and the ideological and value bases of the other disciplines working in mental health practice. To be openly adversarial is to regress to the very win/lose, us/them position which is at the heart of the ontology that we have rejected. Our graduates need to work with both tolerance and understanding in multidisciplinary teams to the point where they are confident of, and comfortable in, making a specific social work contribution.

I have found that this is a challenge which not all students are willing to face. Some fear that in working in hierarchical, institutional health settings, they would be swamped by the dominant paradigm; this insight may, in itself, be useful in preparation for professional practice. Others, however, feel more confident; and most at least recognise the important contribution that the social work profession can make in such settings and are willing to try. Philip Thomas (1997) speaks very eloquently of this need for working together in his chapter titled 'Alienation or integration?', where he discusses the importance of understanding the power dynamics of agencies where psychiatrists work, in order to understand and work together for the benefit of the client.

Fourth, students need to contemplate the implications of a broader ontology of mental health for their own practice, such that they are enabled to incorporate mental health issues as a continuum across a wide range of practice arenas in ways which they might not have previously considered. This process requires in turn a reconsideration of their personal philosophy of practice.

Finally, the curriculum looks at the various roles of social work in the developing community-based mental health services. Students have the opportunity to look at some of the resistances to this process mentioned earlier, and to ponder on ways in which their emerging skills can be used to work with these resistances. Again, a holistic philosophy of practice is important here and opportunities need to be addressed with flexibilty and creativity across the spectrum: support networks; social and therapy groups; housing and employment issues; social action and community education; planning, funding and developing the non-government sector; and sensitive research and practice drawing on the stories of consumers themselves.

From all of this, social workers are well equipped in terms of knowledge and training for their most important role, which in my view is to foster consumer involvement in as many aspects of practice as possible. Without this, they and we have little chance of working together to develop a better society.

REFERENCES

American Psychiatric Association (1994) *Diagnostic and Statistical Manual of Mental Disorders* (DSMIV), 4th edn, American Psychiatric Association, Washington DC.

Bainbridge, L. (1985) 'Taking Psychiatry Out of a Social Work Course', in R. Harris (ed.), *Educating Social Workers*, Association of Teachers in Social Work Education, Leicester

Banton, R., Clifford, P., Frosh, S., Lousada, J. and Rosenthall, J. (1985) *The Politics of Mental Health*, Macmillan, London

Bateson, G. (1973) *Steps to an Ecology of Mind*, Paladin, St Albans

Benhabib, S. (1992) *Situating the Self: Gender, Community & Postmodernism in Contemporary Ethics*, Polity Press, Cambridge

Bradley, B. (1989) *Visions of Infancy*, Polity Press, Cambridge

Broverman, I., Broverman, D., Clarkson, F., Rosenkrantz, P. and Vogel, S. (1970) 'Sex-role Stereotypes and Clinical Judgments of Mental Health', *Journal of Consulting and Clinical Psychology*, vol. 34, no. 1, pp. 1–7

Brown, G. and Harris, T. (1978) *The Social Origins of Depression*, Free Press, New York

Caplan, P. (1995) *They Say You're Crazy: How the World's Most Powerful Psychiatrists Decide Who's Normal*, Addison-Wesley, Reading, Mass.

Cohen, S. (1985) *Visions of Social Control: Crime, Punishment and Classification*, Polity Press, Cambridge

Devereux, G. (1987) *Basic Problems of Ethnopsychiatry*, University of Chicago Press, Chicago

Foucault, M. (1967) *Madness & Civilization: A History of Insanity in the Age of Reason*, Tavistock, London

Freire, P. (1972) *Pedagogy of the Oppressed*, Penguin, Harmondsworth

Fromm, E. (1973) *The Anatomy of Human Destructiveness*, Holt, Rinehart and Winston, New York

Fuller Torrey, E. (1997) *Out of the Shadows: Confronting America's Mental Health Crisis*, John Wiley & Sons, New York

Gramsci, A. (1977) *The Prison Notebooks*, Lawrence & Wishart, London

Hekman, S. (1990) *Gender and Knowledge: Elements of a Postmodern Feminism*, Polity Press, Cambridge

Holmes, P. (1992) *The Inner World Outside: Object Relations Theory and Psychodrama*, Tavistock/Routledge, London

HRSCAA (House of Representative Standing Committee on Aboriginal Affairs) (1979) *Aboriginal Health*, AGPS, Canberra

Human Rights and Equal Opportunity Commission (1993) *Report of the National Enquiry into the Human Rights of People with Mental Illness*, AGPS, Canberra.

Illich, I. (1976) *Limits to Medicine*, M. Boyars, London

Kleinman, A. (1988) *Rethinking Psychiatry: From Cultural Category to Personal Experience*, Free Press, New York

Marshall, R. (1988) 'The Role of Ideology in the Individualization of Distress', *The Psychologist, Bulletin of the British Psychological Society*, vol. 2, pp. 67–69

Mendel, W.M. and Rapport, S. (1969) 'Determinants of the Decision for Psychiatric Hospitalization', *Archives of General Psychiatry*, vol. 20, pp. 321–28

Morice, R. (1978) 'Psychiatric Diagnosis in a Transcultural Setting: The Importance of Lexical Categories', *British Journal of Psychiatry*, vol. 132, pp. 87–95

Rapoport, R.N. (1960) *Community as Doctor: New Perspectives on a Therapeutic Community*, C.C. Thomas, Springfield

Roheim, G. (1930) *Animism, Magic and the Divine King*, Knopf, New York

Said, E. (1995) *Orientalism*, Penguin, London

Sarup, M. (1993) *An Introductory Guide to Post-structuralism and Postmodernism*, Harvester Wheatsheaf, London

Scheff, T.T. (1966) *Being Mentally Ill: A Sociological Theory*, Aldine Publishing Co., Chicago

Thomas, P. (1997) *The Dialectics of Schizophrenia*, Free Association Books, London, New York

Warner, R. (1994) *Recovery from Schizophrenia: Psychiatry and Political Economy*, Routledge and Kegan Paul, New York

Zerbe, K. (1993) *The Body Betrayed: Women, Eating Disorders, and Treatment*, American Psychiatric Press, Inc., Washington DC

13 Critical reflectivity in education and practice
Jan Fook

Critical reflection, as a process and a technique for learning about and improving upon practice, is gaining popularity in social work circles. However, there is a danger that the process may be adopted without a full understanding of its critical possibilities. In this chapter, I attempt to connect the theory and practice of critical reflection with some of the epistemological principles associated with postmodern critical traditions. By identifying and clarifying these connections, I hope to enable social workers and educators to better realise the emancipatory potential of the critical reflection process.

I have designed the chapter, insofar as is possible, to model a reflective process. Thus it begins with accounts from two different social workers, reflecting on aspects of their experiences. I have chosen to begin in this way because my intention is to allow the reflective accounts to speak for themselves, to illustrate the process and power of critical reflection. Later in the chapter, I draw out some salient aspects of the accounts, and connect these features with the process and theory of critical reflection. The following section then traces the ways in which critical reflection is congruent with postmodern critical thinking. Lastly, I end the chapter by reflecting on the process of its construction, and my own experience with critical reflection and postmodern critical thinking.

TWO REFLECTIVE ACCOUNTS

The first account comes from Thelma, a graduating social worker, speaking about a critical incident for which she had sought professional supervision, and felt disillusioned by the outcome.

After the critical incident with the client I reported the case to my supervisor because it involved child protection and I believed she should know the details of the case. The discussion with the supervisor of the critical incident and the ensuing handing back of the client was expected. The unexpected was the tone of the discussion. The interpretation made by the supervisor was that I had pushed the client into divulging too much, thereby allowing the client's power to flow on to me. To have my supervisor (who is known to be one of the foremost supervisors around) say this just stopped me in my tracks. My first reaction influenced what happened next as I did not regain my equilibrium enough to question the initial analysis. This probably allowed her to think her assumption was correct. If I had interpreted the supervisor's analysis as inquisitive questioning rather than an accusation of incompetent practice, the emotional element would have been controllable on my part. I had intended to report in detail what happened and then debrief, but this never happened . . .

A main theme emerging from this session was my inability to assert myself. I allowed my inability to 'name' things to take over, and did not claim my own professional skill base. The language my supervisor used was eloquent, fast and full of comfortable jargon. This is something she is renowned for. I would quite often ask her to qualify her jargon, however in this instance I didn't. In my recently recognised 'victim' mode, I gave up my narrative for hers, just accepted the tabled analysis of the situation and withdrew. My withdrawal had two negative functions: first, it allowed me to indulge in a safe space of 'the victim', therefore I did not have to take a chance in debate; and second, by not extending myself, the supervisor was denied a constructive space where she could mirror her argument. Foucault (cited in Sawicki 1991: 52) claims power is 'exercised rather than possessed . . .' The power I exercised against myself would otherwise be known as sabotage. This demonstrates the fluidity of power: it has so many interpretations, allowing its influence to go unrecognised through biography, therefore hardly ever challenged.

So what is happening is that I am accepting what I regard as inappropriate behaviour from people who hold power over me, and then angrily revisit the site of the 'other's' behaviour, rather than look at why I behave this way. In a sense, this allowed me the power of being the victim with all the moral righteousness on my side. With this covert knowledge I have been able to exclude myself from the equation, as this would be considered 'vicitm blaming', not a socially accepted situation. This behaviour of mine has been carried through with each interaction I have viewed as wrongfully confronting.

I find Thelma's account striking in its humility: her ability to recognise how her own interpretations and behaviour may have played a role in her own 'sabotage'. Yet she is able to transcend the potential humiliation of this realisation, to theorise her experience with the more formalised theory of Foucault, and, in so doing, to build for herself a broader, more generalised theory about her own behaviour in similar situations.

Some of these themes are also evident in the second account, from Amy Rossiter, a social work academic and educator from York University, Toronto, Canada. Amy is reflecting on what she terms 'curriculum transformation—the attempt to deal with systemic inequality as it is manifested in educational process and content' (Rossiter 1995: 5).

In my case, as a white, Western woman, I could not get to the starting line of curriculum transformation until I had challenged my notion of society as made up of racists and non-racists, in which I was in the non-racist category, condemning racists who were spoiling things for people of colour. I recall my surprise several years ago, when, at the end of a feminist theory course I had taken, two black women from the Caribbean announced that the feminist theory 'we' had been studying with great enthusiasm had nothing to do with their experience. They described their connections with their families, their relationships to their mothers, grandmothers and aunts, and they described the place of racism in their lives. I felt stunned and shocked that the idea that the feminist theory I felt was so necessary in explaining my life did not have the same explanatory power because their life circumstances were different. I did not move very far with that recognition, however. The problem was somehow 'out there', not really part of my orbit. A curiosity, really, that feminism didn't seem to fit some women.

Glimmers of the connection between my identity and curriculum transformation first occurred to me when I was working with a collective of feminist practitioners. There was a woman of colour in the group. She occasionally would bring up issues relating to immigrant women, or clients who are people of colour. The rest of us would listen politely and nod our heads in agreement and resume the white women's agenda, and wish her luck with her issues. It was rather shocking to discover after some months of unquestioned camaraderie that she didn't feel part of the group. I did not understand this at all. I felt she was a friend, so what was the problem? The problem, as I gradually learned, was my failure to realise that it made a difference that she was a person of colour in a white group. That I had made her up to be as white as the rest of us, and she found that offensive. That we left the issues of race and ethnicity up to her. That, in the final analysis, I had not understood that the devaluation of people through race created a deep division between her and me: a division that couldn't be transcended by friendship.

Part of the work that I have been trying to do involves answering the question: 'How could I not have known that racism could separate me from my friend?' I have found that the partial answers take me back to my history, and that that exploration continues to create more questions about my present and future from each partial answer about the past. Indeed, the hardest part of the work has been accepting how deeply questions of both identity and knowledge are called up in the process of curriculum transformation, and that there will be no finished place for identity in a racist present.' (Rossiter 1995: 7–8)

FEATURES OF THE CRITICALLY REFLECTIVE PROCESS

What are the common themes in these two accounts? First, both women place themselves directly in the situation—this is done in a number of ways. For example, Thelma notes the influence of herself on the situation by recognising how both *her own personal reactions* and *interpretations* might have influenced the supervisor's reactions:

> My first reaction influenced what happened next as I did not regain my equilibrium enough to question the initial analysis. This probably allowed her to think her assumption was correct. If I had interpreted the supervisor's analysis as inquisitive questioning rather than an accusation of incompetent practice, the emotional element would have been controllable on my part.

Amy recognises the influence of self through locating her *social and cultural background* as a 'white, Western woman'. Her reflections on her reactions also lead her to analyse the role of her own *history* in her present thinking.

Both Amy and Thelma also note the role of their own *emotions*: Thelma her anger and Amy her shock. Another striking element of all accounts is the humility, the non-dogmatic nature, of their thinking. Each person owns their ideas and assumptions as being particular to them, yet nevertheless generalisable, in an inductive way, to broader learning for themselves.

Amy acknowledges the role of her *own assumptions*. For example, the assumption that friendship could transcend issues of race actually blinded her, she felt, to issues of race and the different experiences engendered from it.

Reflectivity, as embodied in these accounts, involves the ability to locate oneself in a situation through the recognition of how actions and interpretations, social and cultural background and personal history, emotional aspects of experience, and personally held assumptions and values influence the situation.

What is even more interesting, on another level, is how the location of themselves in the situation, whilst strikingly humbling (particularly in Thelma's and Amy's cases), is actually experienced as potentially empowering, rather than 'victim-blaming'. Thelma's reflections led her to an analysis which allows her to identify a past disempowering trend to take a passive 'victim' stance. Amy's reflections led her to recognise how questions of identity must be confronted in order to undertake the process of curriculum transformation. It is as if both people, in being able to recognise their own influence in the situation, are able to locate a concrete site for change.

We might term this aspect of reflectivity a type of *responsibility*, an ability to recognise personal influence and to develop a *sense of agency* in a situation. However, with this sense of agency, it is notable that each person integrates, in a very interwoven and easy way, analysis with action, personal experience with political awareness and macro and micro analyses. Personal background and assumptions are linked with broader received wisdoms and, similarly, personal and concrete experiences act as a springboard to broaden thinking.

Thelma links her own observations with Foucauldian notions of power, and is able to uncover, and question, a victim-blaming, potentially sabotaging influence in her approach to people who are more powerful than her.

Amy uncovers covert assumptions about divisions between racist and non-racist people, and a tendency to blame the racists, until she recognised how her own assumptions could also be racist in their very denial of racist issues. By putting the problem 'out there', she was denying her own participation in supporting ideologies (such as feminism) which perpetuated racism.

Whilst the *capacity for questioning and change* emerges as a hopeful theme, so does the glimmer of *uncertainty*. This is most evident in Amy's account. Amy speaks of an ongoing process in which questions throw up further questions, and suggests that 'there will be no finished place for identity in a racist present'.

By way of summary, the two accounts illustrate a number of features of the critically reflective process. First, the ability to acknowledge and appreciate the influence of self (personal reactions—behavioural and emotional, interpretations, social and cultural background, personal history or experience) in determining and changing a situation is paramount. Second, the recognition of personally held, often hidden or unconscious assumptions, and their role in influencing a situation, is also crucial. Third, a sense of responsibility, of agency, an appreciation of how each player can act upon to influence a situation, is evident. Coupled with this is an ability to interweave analysis with action, to engage in a process of inductive and creative thinking, so that specific personal experiences act as a springboard to broaden understanding. Lastly, a capacity to question, to tolerate uncertainty, and to utilise this as a catalyst for active change, seems to develop.

We have extrapolated these features from an analysis of the two reflective accounts. But how do these features relate to more formalised theories of critical reflection as presented in the literature?

THEORIES OF CRITICAL REFLECTION

I began my chapter deliberately in this way, because I wanted to illustrate, rather than argue for, the power of critical reflection. I now want to outline these points in more detail.

Critical reflection is not necessarily the same as reflection. There is a danger that the idea of reflection can become an orthodoxy, a catch-all phrase diluted to mean any type of 'thinking about' a situation.

The reflective approach is probably most attributed to the work of Argyris and Schon (1976) and Schon (1983, 1987). It has more latterly been picked up by social work educators such as Papell and Skolnik (1992) and Gould and Taylor (1996). The reflective approach is based on a questioning of the usefulness of traditional approaches to knowledge-building for professionals, since traditional approaches seem to result in a disjuncture between the 'theory' and the 'practice' of professionals. Traditional approaches to knowledge building and knowledge use assume an empirial approach—that is, that knowledge is generated objectively, and that generalised theories are developed by researching phenomena in a scientific manner. Practitioners are then presumed to use this knowledge in a deductive way, applying general theory to act in specific situations. Alternatively, a reflective approach sees theory as being implicit in actions, which therefore may or may not be consistent with the generalised theory a practitioner believes themselves to be acting upon. This is a more inductive process, in which practice theory is developed out of the everyday experience of professionals. A reflective approach therefore questions the positivist assumptions of a traditional approach. Reflective approaches also emphasise the intuition and artistry involved in professional practice, and the importance of context and interpretation in influencing action. Reflective approaches to learning generally rely on experiential methods.

If we refer back to the three accounts quoted earlier, we see that each person engages in a process of theory-building by reflecting on their own practice. Thelma develops a theory about how and why some of her own self-protective behaviour contributes to her own 'sabotage', and is able to extend aspects of Foucault's concept of power through this. Amy is engaged in developing a theory of curriculum transformation, through her realisation of the inextricability of identity in confronting issues of race.

Critical approaches to knowledge generation arise out of a critical social science tradition (Carr and Kemmis 1986). The main features of this tradition (Agger 1991) are based on a recognition that capitalist social structures are perpetuated through the operation of a type of 'false consciousness', in that members of society are unaware that present social structures and relations are constructed and therefore transformable. Existing arrangements are maintained partly through external exploitation, and partly through a form of self-deception. A critical approach is therefore wary of positivism as the accepted form of knowledge generation, since it fosters alienation, or the experience of being distanced from the capacity to change the situation. Thus it is crucial, in a critical approach, to develop a consciousness which is able to imagine the transformability of current arrangements. This means it is necessary to be able to distinguish between knowledge which is generated empirically, and that which is generated through self-reflection and interaction. This combination of knowledge is known as reconstructed historical materialism (Agger 1991, summarising Habermas). Because there is a recognition that this combination of knowledge is necessary, then processes of communication, dialogue and reflection become important in generating this knowledge. One of the main features of a critical approach, then, is the emancipatory element—the capacity to question and change existing power relations. A second main feature is the interactive way in which such emancipatory knowledge is developed.

Reflective and critical approaches therefore share some common features: a critique of positivism; a recognition of reflective ways of knowing; and a reliance on interactional processes in the generation of this knowledge. However, what is also vital to a critical approach—which is not necessarily articulated in a reflective stance— is the *emancipatory* project, the capacity to analyse social situations and to transform social relations on the basis of this analysis; and to combine this analysis with self-reflective knowledge.

Brookfield (1995), in discussing teaching practice, points up the differences between reflection and critical reflection more succinctly. In his view, the reflective process is about 'hunting assumptions' (1995: 2), paradigmatic, prescriptive and causal. But:

> Reflection is not, by definition, critical . . . reflection becomes critical when it has two distinctive purposes. The first is to understand how considerations of power undergird, frame, and distort educational processes and interactions. The second is to question assumptions and practices that seem to make our teaching lives easier but actually work against our own best long term interests. (1995: 8)

Thus, according to Brookfield, it is the ability to uncover thinking (assumptions) which contributes to constructed power relations, and is self-defeating because of its incompatability with espoused desirable goals, which marks critical reflection from reflection.

A critically reflective approach therefore relies upon knowledge which is generated both empirically and self-reflectively, and in a process of interaction, in order to analyse, resist and change constructed power relations, structures and ways of thinking. Both accounts, from Thelma and Amy, are *reflective*, in that each connects her own experience and thinking with 'received' theories or wisdoms; and each analyses, and in some cases modifies, these theories through this process of reflective connections. But Thelma and Amy are also *critically reflective*. in that each also constructs a theory as a basis for changing existing power relations in their respective situations.

HOW DOES CRITICAL REFLECTION RELATE TO POSTMODERN CRITICAL THEORY?

There are many similarities between critical social science and postmodernism and poststructuralism (Kellner and Best 1991: 215), and a significant number of social theorists have developed what is now being termed a postmodern critical approach. Some writers are now developing the similarities between the two as the basis for a new critical approach in social work (Rossiter 1996; Leonard 1997).

The parameters of postmodern critical theory have been outlined in the beginning chapters. By way of summary here, a postmodern perspective or way of theorising pays attention to the ways in which social relations and structures are constructed, particularly to the ways in which language, narrative and discourses shape power relations and our understanding of them. In particular, dominant structures are subject to question because of the ways in which meanings are constructed on oppositional lines (therefore defining difference, and often devaluing it, in relation to a dominant group), multiple perspectives are silenced or marginalised, and a unified, or logocentric, view of 'truth' is perpetuated. Also in question is a 'linear' and cumulative path to understanding; therefore the changing and contextual nature of meaning and identity is also emphasised. A postmodern analysis therefore involves a 'deconstruction' of constructed meanings, in order to uncover hidden or multiple perspectives, and dominant discourses and the power relations they support. A postmodern critical perspective emphasises the emancipatory possibilities of a postmodern analysis, the possibilities for challenging, resisting and changing dominant power structures which are uncovered by deconstruction.

Critical reflection is integral to a postmodern critical perspective in a number of ways. First, it is valued as a way of knowing, since it constitutes an alternative to dominant 'logocentric' purely positivistic and empiricist approaches to discovery. With a basis in personal and concrete experience, it opens the way for the perspectives of marginalised groups (for example, the practitioner and the student) to be valued and developed; and it opens the way for marginalised aspects of experience to be incorporated into understandings of the world (for example, the emotions and personal history). Second, it is valued as a process, because of the emphasis on interaction, communication, change and uncertainty inherent in it. In the process of critical reflection, you are forced to pay attention to interactive aspects of situations (your own influence on the situation—interpretations, behaviour, hidden assumptions), and how this influence might have affected power relations or perpetuated existing structures and thinking. The accounts we opened with each illustrate how Amy and Thelma entered into a type of dialogue with themselves, engaging in a round of questioning and rethinking their own behaviour and assumptions, and connections with their personal history and context.

Third, because a process of critical reflection allows a person to make connections between concrete experience, broader theorising, and specific context, it more easily allows the person to locate a clear site for change—because the analysis is contextual and of concrete experience, so are the possibilities for change. There is thus a more direct, and actionable, relationship between analysis and practice. Theorising, and the development of models and strategies for practice, becomes part of the domain of the practising worker, rather than necessarily only that of the academic researcher. Barriers, and the related inherent power relations, are thus broken down.

REFLECTIONS

I pride myself on being an efficient writer, but I have struggled and agonised over the construction of this chapter with much more than my usual efforts. Initially, it was to be simply a chapter in which I set out my arguments for the similarities between critical reflection and postmodern critical theory. I already had the similarities in my head, and felt I was clear about them, so knew that this would not take too much time.

What has been difficult is the dawning realisation that I could not write about a reflective approach in a traditional didactic manner. From a poststructural stance, it was clear that the form, process and manner of my expression had to be an effective and appropriate vehicle for communicating my ideas about critical reflectivity. I searched for a way, a non-dogmatic way, which would allow the approach to speak for itself, so that you the reader would gain insights from your own reflection on the material, rather than relying on being convinced by the force of my intellectual argument.

This chapter, then, also represents an exercise in demonstrating and illustrating (rather than intellectually arguing for) a reflective process. I began with the experience of two social workers, told in their own words. I then went on to reflect on their accounts in terms of their similarities. I then drew out the points of connection between their accounts and the more formalised 'textbook' theory around reflectivity, critical approaches and postmodernism. What I finish with here is a reflection on this chapter, with some further questions about what thinking needs further development in order to effect some change on the basis of these reflections.

A common reaction that I have found to a reflective way of writing and thinking is dismay, and sometimes a dismissive discrediting. People regard it as 'unacademic' to write in a personal way, and certainly 'lightweight' to write in what appears to be a descriptive style. The hidden assumption appears to be that, if it is easy, it can't be good! (And also if something is personal, it is by definition unacademic, and therefore of limited value.) I must say I find these assumptions, particularly the latter ones, quite disturbing in a profession like social work which espouses the value of experience (presumably only that of our service users, not that of workers). In selecting and reflecting upon the accounts at the beginning of this chapter, I would have to say they are anything but easy, and certainly not lightweight. Although written in a highly personal and descriptive manner, they are redolent with analysis, with theorising, with creative connections and original insights, with difficult emotions and realisations—moreover, with ideas which have the capacity to change constructed ways of thinking and acting.

Another common reaction to postmodernism and to a reflective approach, is fear and criticism of a perceived relativism, as if somehow postmodernists must give up a stable set of values and then flap aimlessly about in the wind. There is also the accusation that there is an implied political neutrality in postmodernism, which leaves its exponents open to political corruption (as if those with more certainly espoused political left-wing views are not open to corruption or co-option). To what extent are these types of thinking themselves examples of modernist constructions? Does a set of values—social justice or otherwise—exist without a particular expression in a particular situation? Even my 'absolutist' description of social justice in 1998 must be rooted in the language and battles of a particular context.

I wonder if it is actually modernist constructions of ideas and sets of political ideas which see these as having a life of their own, as anthropomorphic constructions which have a type of supra-identity, over and above the human beings and social conditions which have created them. In many ways it may be these modernist types of thinking, these ways of constructing ideas and our relationships to them, from which our criticisms arise.

In addition, to place too much importance on the differences between modernist and postmodernist thinking may be to miss the bigger picture. As Kellner and Best (1991: 257) point out, there is a tradition (Marx, Dewey, Weber) within modernist theory which shares similarities with postmodern thinking, in that it is non-dogmatic, open to disconfirmation and revision, reflexive and self-critical, and thus eschews 'the quest for certainty, foundations and universal laws'.

> the best modern social theorists recognize the differentiation and fragmentation within modernity, while also providing a language that addresses its integrative and macroscopic features . . . the task of social theory is . . . to provide original and illuminating perspectives that call attention to new phenomona, that disclose relationships hitherto obscured, or that even provide new ways of seeing . . . (1991: 258, 270)

It is, however, possible to take on the epistemological aspects of postmodernism, to take on a doubtful and deconstructive stance in relation to discourses, to constructed thinking and arrangements; yet to aim, with this sceptical stance and process, to analyse and criticise current arrangements in terms of their inequitable and oppressive power relations. Thus postmodern critical theory is clear on process and values, but uncertain about specific expressions and strategies—these latter will be determined by place, time, players and context.

What is difficult and challenging about postmodern critical theory is embodied in these reflections for me. In my experience, the challenge of postmodernism is not so much the uncertainty it entails, but the very radical change in forms of thinking and expression, in accepted notions of standards of academic theorising, in accepted methods of teaching, in accepted ways of establishing professional authority—indeed, in all the accepted ways of maintaining existing power relations. We are all implicated in these processes, as Amy Rossiter so poignantly discovered. Postmodern critical theory and the critically reflective thinking it entails are never easy, because one's accepted notions about what is acceptable are always open to question, and the less open they are, the more painful they are to unearth. For me, taking on a postmodern critical stance means I have not joined a club which tells me the right ideas to espouse, and lets me feel comfortable in the safe confines of the company of like-minded people. Rather, I feel I have begun to engage in a process which ought constantly to keep me honest, and certainly keeps me forever humble, and forever vigilant, about how over-certainty can blind me to other, new and maybe better perspectives.

CONCLUDING QUESTIONS AND UNCERTAINTIES

Is there room, then, for critical reflection in the practice of the professional social worker, confronted with increasing managerial control and an accompanying deprofessionalisation and a technocratisation of skills? If critical reflection is indeed about a process, about a way in which we engage with our contexts in order to deconstruct and critically reconstruct, then it is likely all the more necessary in the current climate. Critical reflection should allow us to not take anything for granted, to actually re-analyse situations in ways which will allow new actions, and to change power relations at both macro and micro levels. In a way, it is an attitude, an approach, rather than a set of new skills. What it does do is allow that possibilities and sites for resistance and change will be newly created, and that new strategies and skills may arise out of these.

Let us return to our two social workers. Thelma will, at the very least, no longer participate in her own sabotage, but will be better equipped to engage with more powerful people on a more equal footing. And Amy will continue to develop courses which are more cross-culturally appropriate and racially relevant, courses which should be more relevant and effective across a range of diverse populations.

It is easy to become alarmed at the increasing managerial controls on professional autonomy, and to assume that we will be forced to engage in a more routinised practice as the future of our profession. However, I would argue that, in a managerialist culture, there is perhaps a greater need for the articulation of professional skills and knowledge, for the accountability of professional practice, and for the research and development of the practice of professional practitioners. And, whilst there is a place for the better understanding of professional practice, there will be a place for reflective learning, for better integrating the theory and practice of our professional experience. Jones and Jordan (1996: 267) put the issue succinctly:

> The real integration between theory and practice will come not from a ponderous, rigid body of knowledge, but from the humility to learn from practitioners' experiences.

This is the major contribution of a critical reflective approach to practice.

REFERENCES

Agger, B. (1991) 'Critical Theory, Poststructuralism, Postmodernism: Their Sociological Relevance', *Annual Review of Sociology*, vol. 17, pp. 105–31

Argyris, C. and Schon, D. (1976) *Theory in Practice: Increasing Professional Effectiveness*, Jossey-Bass, San Francisco

Brookfield, S.D. (1995) *Becoming a Critically Reflective Teacher*, Jossey-Bass, San Francisco

Carr, W. and Kemmis, S. (1986) *Becoming Critical: Education, Knowledge and Action Research*, Deakin University Press, Geelong

Jones, M. and Jordan, B. (1996) 'Knowledge and Practice in Social Work', in M. Preston-Shoot (ed.), *Social Work Education in a Changing Policy Context*, Whiting & Birch, London

Gould, N. and Taylor, I. (1996) *Reflective Learning for Social Work*, Arena, Aldershot

Kellner, D. and Best, S. (1991) *Postmodern Theory: Critical Interrogations*, Guildford, New York

Leonard, P. (1997) *Postmodern Welfare: Reconstructing an Emancipatory Project*, Sage, London

Papell, C.P. and Skolnik, L. (1992) 'The Reflective Practitioner: A Contemporary Paradigm's Significance for Social Work Education', *Journal of Social Work Education*, vol. 28, no. 1, pp. 18–26

Rossiter, A. (1995) 'Entering the Intersection of Identity, Form, and Knowledge: Reflections on Curriculum Transformation', *Canadian Journal of Community Mental Health*, vol. 14, no. 1, pp. 5–14

——(1996) 'A Perspective on Critical Social Work', *Journal of Progressive Human Services*, vol. 7, no. 2, pp. 23–41.

Salmonds, J. (unpublished) Untitled Account

Sawicki, J. (1991) *Disciplining Foucault: Feminism, Power and the Body*, Routledge, New York

Schon, D. (1983) *The Reflective Practitioner*, Basic Books, New York

——(1987) *Educating the Reflective Practitioner*, Jossey-Bass, San Francisco

PART V

Critically interrogating the postmodern

14 Postmodernism, critical theory and social work
Jim Ife

In the current social, economic and political climate of change and instability, many of the older certainties of social work practice no longer seem relevant. The apparently unproblematic commitment to ideals such as human rights and social justice, the idea that empirically verified social science could guide practice, and the assumption of a universalist and prescriptive code of ethics no longer seem to meet the needs of many practitioners. The current practice environment is more uncertain, more hostile, and constantly changing, so that the old certainties do not provide a social worker with the secure basis for practice that might have been the case ten years ago. In such a climate, the 'postmodern' world view has an obvious and understandable appeal, as it seeks to describe a world which is characterised by uncertainty, doubt, relativism, change and constant redefinition of 'reality'. Such a perspective seems likely to be more appropriate for the contemporary social work practitioner. However, at the same time, a lingering doubt remains as to whether it also represents a 'sell-out' to the very ideologies of individualism, greed and exploitation against which social workers have claimed to stand. Additionally, there is a suggestion that postmodernism requires social workers to abandon the values which form the very core of social work practice.

It is certainly true that the current context of practice has shown up the inadequacies of the theory and knowledge bases of social work. The social democratic consensus, grounded in positivist and empirically verified social science, which formed the basis for the development of the welfare state within which social work has been practised and understood, has proved to be theoretically weak, and unable to withstand the strong critiques from neo-conservative, Marxist or anarchist positions. Concepts such as 'core values', 'social justice', 'human rights', 'professional ethics' and 'skilled helper' are no longer uncontroversial, but are now highly problematic. Practitioners, scholars and students, in search of a coherent basis for practice, are therefore seeking alternatives from different paradigms of social science: postmodernism, poststructuralism, feminism, postcolonialism, and so on. It is in this context that the recent interest in postmodernism as a basis for social work practice must be understood. In examining the relevance of postmodernism for social work, the position that will be argued here is that postmodernism is a necessary, but not a sufficient, basis for conceptualising theory and practice.

To generalise about postmodernism is, of course, problematic. There are different strands of postmodernist thinking, most notably the important difference between what Rosenau (1992) describes as *affirmative* and *sceptical* postmodernism. Indeed, to assume that there is one 'right' form of postmodernism would be to contradict one of the basic tenets of a postmodernist position, which allows for and values diversity, and which refuses to accept that there can be only one form of conceptualisation. The generalisations which follow, therefore, must be treated critically, and must be read as representing perhaps one 'ideal type' of postmodernism rather than necessarily encompassing all the strands of postmodernist thought. Indeed, one of the problems with discussing postmodernism is that, simply by using the word, one implies a single definable body of thought, when in reality the very nature of postmodernism rules out such uniformity.

POSTMODERNITY AND POSTMODERNISM

The idea of the postmodern presents both descriptive and normative critiques of contemporary society, both of which are of interest to social work. At the descriptive level (where the term 'post-modernity' rather than 'postmodernism' is normally used), the critique sees society as having moved towards a state which can be described as 'postmodern'. Such a position is argued persuasively by Galtung (1996), who identifies, for the sake of analysis, two forms of social and organisational relations: alpha and beta. These are similar to Tönnies' (1955) well-known categories of Gemeinschaft and Gesellschaft. In Galtung's terms, alpha organisations are large, often hierarchical, and involve a large number of relatively superficial, specific and instrumental relationships between people: we deal with many people in our day-to-day life, but we do not really get to know any of them in a close, intimate or personal way. Beta organisations, on the other hand, have smaller numbers of people interacting in more intensive and multi-functional ways, and their size is necessarily limited by their intensity. Where Galtung differs from Tönnies and other classical sociologists is that, rather than seeing a simple transition from one kind of society to another (beta to alpha), he suggests that both can occur at once—there can be strong beta organisations existing within strong alpha organisations. Examples might be a strong friendship (beta) group within a large corporation (alpha), a close-knit church community (beta) within a city (alpha), and so on. For Galtung, there is value in both alpha and beta. We need alpha organisations for material development, progress and to provide us with the kind of lifestyle we have come to expect. We also need beta organisations for our personal nurturing, feeling of belonging, need for community, and so on. Galtung traces historical development through four stages. The first is *primitive societies*, where beta was strong but alpha was weak. This allowed for personal and social development, but not for high levels of technological and economic development. His second stage is *traditional societies*, where strong alpha organisation developed alongside strong beta, allowing for both social and economic development. Large-scale social structures (usually hierarchical) emerged in different civilisations, and added a new dimension to the human experience. His third stage of historical change, *modern societies*, sees the decline of beta organisations while strong alpha organisations are maintained; this is the loss of community experienced over the last two centuries as a result of the forces of modernisation and capitalism. In this stage, of course, the welfare state (made up of alpha organisations) became necessary in order to meet those personal needs which were no longer met by the weakening beta structures of family and community. Galtung then suggests that we are now moving into a fourth stage, postmodern societies, where alpha structures too break down, where people feel increasingly alienated by social organisations, and where increasing numbers are marginalised or excluded. In this, Galtung is echoing the sentiments of the more pessimistic of the postmodernists, who claim that we are entering a world which, far from being united in a global vision of humanity and a single internationalist identity, is increasingly fragmented and differentiated, with weak social structures and with fractured relativism becoming the dominant paradigm.

In this analysis, Galtung represents the descriptive form of postmodern writing. He is describing what is happening in society, in the tradition of the detached social scientist. He does not necessarily welcome the transition to postmodernity; indeed, he makes it clear that he views it with alarm and dismay. However, he presents the postmodern age as something which is developing, whether we like it or not, and as requiring an appropriate response from people like social workers.

The normative view of postmodernism (as opposed to postmodernity) sees a postmodern perspective as a useful way to view the world, suggesting that it opens up new possibilities for understanding and for action. It sees the conventional positivist world view, based in enlightenment thinking, as increasingly irrelevant, and advocates a new paradigm based on the valuing of difference, multiple realities and the 'death of the meta-narrative'. While the descriptive perspective is concerned with identifying and accepting an important historical transition, the normative perspective is concerned also with advocating an alternative world view, or 'paradigm shift'.

A number of writers and commentators seek to maintain an essentially modernist paradigm while trying to understand the postmodern world from a more descriptive perspective. Indeed, this is the position of writers such as Galtung, who is concerned to understand the postmodern world but does not adopt the postmodernism's assumptions about the nature of knowledge and of reality (i.e. the postmodern 'paradigm'). Galtung's position represents a minimal postmodern position for social work. It is essential that social workers understand that the age of modernist certainty is over, and that we are now entering a period characterised by a lack of predictability and permanency, by weak and transitory structures, and by alternatives being constantly deconstructed and reconstructed within a context of fragmentation and difference. Trying to understand this from within an essentially modernist paradigm is fairly common in conventional social science and political discourse. It is characterised by the phrases 'a rapidly changing world', 'managing change' and the popular oxymoron 'planning for uncertainty'. This acknowledgment of the reality of postmodernity, while discounting a postmodernist paradigm as a means for understanding it, is perhaps a form of postmodern thought with which social workers are most comfortable.

Such a position, by trying to understand postmodernism from within a modernist world view, is essentially contradictory. In a postmodern society, it is surely inconsistent to reject a postmodern perspective in attempting to understand 'reality', and in seeking a justification for human action. To do so is to distance the observer from the subject of the observation, and such a separation, while characteristic of an objectivist or positivist paradigm, is incompatible with postmodernity. In a postmodern world, it is in the constant acts of deconstruction and reconstruction that meaning is derived, rather than through detached scientific observation, and hence the social scientist or social worker cannot be separated from the object of study. To some degree, it is therefore necessary for a social worker or social researcher to adopt a postmodern paradigm in order to understand a postmodern world.

PROBLEMS OF POSTMODERNISM

A complete and uncritical adoption of a postmodernist stance, however, raises problems for social workers. These problems stem from postmodernism's rejection of the 'meta-narrative', in favour of relativism. Social work, in its commitment to something called 'social justice' and its insistence on a core value component for the profession, is grounded in meta-narratives, whether they be traditional commitments such as 'the inherent worth of the individual' or more structural positions informed by an analysis of class, gender and race, and an understanding of counter-oppressive practice. The very idea of 'counter-oppressive' social work assumes a meta-narrative of oppression, and hence to deny the meta-narrative is to deny much of what social work has traditionally held to be central to its practice.

The impact of thereby weakening the meta-narratives of social justice, in the current political climate, is substantial and alarming. While academic discourse may celebrate the death of the meta-narrative and the emergence of multiple realities, the world of social work practice is confronted with a meta-narrative of frightening power, and with the imposition of a single reality which denies the very basis of social work. The orthodoxy of economic rationalism, managerialism, neo-conservative economics, blind faith in deregulation, market forces and a minimal role for the state remains largely unchallenged within the dominant public discourse, and a concentration on postmodernism has resulted in those practitioners who would oppose the dominant ideology being largely denied the intellectual tools to provide a sustained critique and to advocate an alternative. Indeed, it can be suggested that the simultaneous rise of neo-conservative ideology and postmodernist thinking is no coincidence; postmodernism is a very convenient framework for the legitimation of 'market forces' and for the erosion of a strong public sector. For the left to be spending its energies on analysing and deconstructing discourses of power, praising relativism and claiming that the era of unified visions of social justice is past, often in extremely inaccessible language, is very convenient for those who wish to pursue an ideology of greed, selfishness, increased inequality and a denial of human rights in the interests of free markets and private profit. It seems characteristic of the intellectual left to retreat into scholasticism when a program of action is not clearly evident, and at a time when neo-conservative ideology reigns largely unchallenged in the public arena, it is unfortunate that so much of the energy of those seeking an alternative is taken up with arcane debates about the finer points of postmodernist philosophy. In this way, the intellectual left seems to provide little help for those concerned with actually trying to do something about making the world a better place, and for those like social workers for whom action, or practice, must be as important as theory.

Nowhere can this be seen more clearly than in the human rights arena. The postmodern scepticism of any universal principles, or meta-narratives, has led to more relativist constructions of human rights, and a corresponding erosion of the idea of human rights being fundamental to all people regardless of culture, nationality, gender, race or whatever. This has not been helpful to human rights activists (including social workers) seeking to protect the basic civil, political, economic, social, cultural and environmental rights of vulnerable individuals, communities and populations. Not many years ago, a strong position advocating human rights went virtually unquestioned, and could represent a solid and comfortable position on which to base social work practice. This is no longer the case, with governments becoming increasingly equivocal on human rights matters, with international human rights treaties being treated with suspicion, and with the increasingly popular view that human rights are somehow relative, and apply differently in different locations. This argument has some understandable appeal to people who wish to be culturally sensitive and culturally appropriate (Galtung 1994), but it is also used to justify the oppression of minorities in places such as Tibet and East Timor, the maintenance of low wages and poor working conditions, the suppression of trade unions and any struggle for workers' rights, the suppression of any form of political dissent, the mutilation of women's bodies, execution of minor criminals, imprisonment without fair trial, ethnic cleansing and the perpetuation of rape, domestic violence, child slavery, and almost any other human rights abuse one could think of. When cultural sensitivities and the advocacy of postmodernist relativism become the excuse not to intervene to seek an end to such practices, and where the work of human rights activists is eroded by intellectual doubt induced by postmodernist uncertainty, it is time to ask serious questions about the appropriateness of the postmodern paradigm in the contemporary world. Postmodernism may be exciting and stimulating at an intellectual level, but it is often not seen as very helpful for practitioners or activists.

POSTMODERNISM AND SOCIAL WORK

It is necessary, therefore, for social workers to retain some kind of universal vision, while at the same time accepting the significant and legitimate contribution of postmodern thinking. The task is to continue to value difference and to reject the imposition of artificial uniformity while maintaining some understanding of universal human values. Postmodernism need not be, and in reality cannot be, an 'all or nothing' choice for social workers. It is rather a case of deciding what contribution postmodernist thought can make to social work, and juxtaposing this with some form of universal framework.

One way in which this can be achieved is through a concentration on process. While a universalist vision may be seen as inappropriate in the sense of an ultimate goal for human action (the humanist project), postmodernism can encourage a concentration on processes—on how we get there rather than on where we are going. Bauman's (1993) treatment of 'postmodern ethics' is perhaps the most significant argument in this direction. Bauman argues that the great moral concerns of modernity—justice, human rights, equity, etc.—are still relevant in a postmodern age; it is the way in which they are understood that must change, rather than the moral concern itself. This leads Bauman to a discussion of ethics as the way in which moral principles, while stripped of their objective universalist claims, can still be important in the making of day-to-day decisions.

Other writers have sought to show that an embracing of the postmodernism need not necessarily negate the structural analysis on which social workers' claims to a social justice foundation rest. Perhaps the most significant has been Peter Leonard (1997), who argues the central importance of a class analysis in understanding contemporary social and economic phenomena, and seeks to blend this with an acceptance of the postmodernist critique and its deconstruction of the familiar social justice discourses of social work, seeing these as being grounded in the discourses of dominant or oppressive groups: Western, male and ruling class. It is through such arguments that a postmodernist valuing of difference and embracing of relativism can be seen as not necessarily contradicting a commitment to social justice and human rights. Indeed it is precisely in the valuing of difference that social justice principles can often be realised; this is the strong message from much feminist and post-colonialist writing. Such a stance, however, does not necessarily deny the validity of some universalist notions of human rights and social justice, and this too is a theme in much of the literature on human emancipation.

Elsewhere (Ife 1997), I have argued that one way in which both universalist visions and the valuing of difference can be held in conjunction is through a discourse of human rights and human needs. From this perspective, human rights are understood as universals. They relate to the things that bind people together as human beings, and transcend culture, race, gender, age, religion and so on. They are the common claims of all humans—who, after all, are the same biological species. One of the problems with much sociological analysis is that it has, necessarily and importantly, concentrated on the things that divide people— gender, race, culture, class, etc.—and has therefore undervalued the things that unite them, namely their common humanity. It can be argued that if we are to live successfully in peace within the ecological limits of this planet, discourses of common humanity must also be emphasised, alongside discourses which emphasise difference and conflict.

The difficulty with such a position, of course, is that attempts to define a common humanity have been influenced largely by Western, male and individualist constructions of 'the nature of man'. Hence the term 'humanist' has become so identified with the Western tradition and the enlightenment that it has excluded or marginalised other perspectives, and the postmodernist, feminist and postcolonialist critiques rightly condemn the 'humanist project' as being essentially oppressive (Carroll 1993). This, however, should not be used to deny the possibility, desirability or necessity of pursuing a vision of common humanity; the task, rather, is to deconstruct traditional humanism and seek its reconstruction in a more inclusive and dialogical process. The idea of universal human rights—the things which every person has a right to expect, regardless of who they are or where they live, by virtue of their very humanity—can provide a space in which such dialogue can take place. It may be true that the current understanding of universal human rights has been unduly influenced by a Western world view, but this is not of itself a sufficient reason for abandoning the whole idea of universal human rights; rather, it requires that we engage in a dialogue about how the idea might be more appropriately reconstructed. The vision of a common universalist humanity has inspired many of the most significant movements for global justice, and to reject such a vision is to reject a powerful impetus for progressive social change.

This universalism in a discourse of human rights can be counterbalanced by a relativism in the discourse of human needs. Statements of need imply an underpinning of rights, but it is in statements of need that those rights are contextualised within particular cultures and environments. The idea of a universal right to education, for example, can result in very different definitions of what is 'needed' in different contexts for that right to be realised. Similarly, rights to freedom of speech, to work, to personal safety and to a healthy physical environment will be expressed as very different 'needs' in different cultural and political contexts. Seeking to universalise needs, beyond the limited definition of basic needs used by Doyal and Gough (1991) can become the ultimate in imposition of an oppressive reality on vulnerable populations, whereas allowing for a relativity of needs within a strong framework of universal rights can enhance the diversity which postmodernism seeks to value, while retaining universal commitments to social justice and human rights.

CRITICAL THEORY AND SOCIAL WORK

Such a formulation goes beyond the confines of a purely postmodernist position as understood by most writers. It requires that both an exclusive modernist universalism and an exclusive postmodern relativism be rejected. Rather, it is necessary to hold both a universalist position based on a reconstruction of humanism, and a relativist position which values (indeed celebrates) difference and which allows for diversity in the way in which human aspirations are expressed and realised. The paradigm within which this can best be achieved is critical theory. There are many varieties of critical theory (Ray 1993), just as there are different varieties of postmodernism, and it can be questioned whether in fact critical theory and postmodernism are necessarily incompatible paradigms. A narrow 'sceptical' interpretation of postmodernism, which discounts any attempt at deriving universal discourses as merely another 'meta-narrative', must be incompatible with critical theory, as critical theory allows for some universal understandings of such ideas as human rights, social justice and oppression. On the other hand, a less ambitious and more affirmative postmodernism may be regarded as compatible with critical theory, in emphasising the importance of context and difference, in seeking ways to inform action, and in its rejection of positivist certainty which is a common feature of both critical theory and postmodernism. Critical theory can readily accept such a version of postmodernism, and the form of critical theory advocated here is one which is informed by, and incorporates, significant elements of a postmodernist position.

The particular value of critical theory is that it values subjective experience, and hence affirms difference and the continual reconstruction of 'reality', while at the same time embedding this within a more macro analysis of structural disadvantage, or oppression. It is in the holding of these two apparently opposing positions, and in seeking to resolve that dialectic, that critical theory both poses intellectual challenges for social workers and others, but also suggests courses of action (or praxis) within the context of the uncertainty, fragmentation and ambiguity of a postmodern world. There are certain aspects of the critical theory paradigm which are of particular significance for social workers, and these will now be briefly explored.

The first is the specific linking of theory and practice. One of the weaknesses of postmodernism for social workers is that it has often concentrated on theorising and has had little to say about actual practice. Such a position may be acceptable for an academic scholar who only has to satisfy the reader of a book or journal, but is of little use for a social worker caught in the reality of day-to-day practice within the crumbling remains of the welfare state, who has to balance the conflicting demands of clients, families, employers and communities in a hostile political context, while seeking to retain some degree of professional integrity, personal life and simple sanity. For such a worker, it is not enough simply to talk about deconstruction and fragmentation; the worker wants some help as to what they might actually do. Critical theory specifically seeks to link theory and practice, through an under-standing of 'praxis', suggesting that one cannot 'do' theory or practice in isolation; rather, it is a reflexive process of learning by doing and of doing by learning. Unless knowledge has some form of practical utility, in helping people to articulate their needs and work towards having them met, it is not particularly important. Critical theory insists that theory be grounded in practice, and vice versa, and so is of particular importance for social workers, who are inevitably concerned with action as well as with understanding.

Critical theory, unlike the positivist paradigm which grew out of the enlightenment and which is quintessentially modernist, accepts the inevitability—and indeed the desirability—of social science being essentially normative. Theory and practice are about trying to achieve particular normative outcomes, cast in the lan-guage of social justice. They are about freedom from oppression, struggles for liberation, and inevitably contain some notion of a just and fair society (specifically rejected by many postmodernist writers). Critical theory can thus re-legitimise a humanist vision—though, as was argued above, this must be reconstructed so as to avoid the ethnocentric, gendered and imperialistic assumptions of conventional Western humanism.

Critical theory also makes specific the important link between the personal and the political. Social work has struggled with the way in which the two are conventionally conceptualised separately, and the history of social work reflects the split between 'macro' and 'micro' practice. The very fact that social workers have been concerned with how the two might be related indicates how the dominant paradigm has required their separate conceptualisation. For critical theory, however, there can be no separation of the two. Praxis must occur across both the personal and the political. In this sense, again, critical theory is more relevant for social work than postmodernism, as postmodernism has generally been inadequate in dealing with the larger political/structural issues. Indeed, the inherently apolitical nature of much postmodernist writing has led to the criticism, mentioned above, of postmodernism as reflecting an essentially neo-liberal ideology, and as providing comfort to those who seek to justify a social system based on inequality and individualism. Such a position is incompatible with the values of social work as understood by many social workers.

Critical theory thus allows, and specifically encourages, the holding of apparently contradictory opposites: theory and practice, personal and political, etc. It requires a dialectical perspective which suggests that it is from the tensions between these apparent contradictions that creative change can emerge. This is also based on a questioning of the dualistic thinking which is inherent in much traditional social science and social work literature. Feminist writers such as Plumwood (1993) have been influential in suggesting that the way in which we have tended to construct dualisms has not only reflected a patriarchal world view, but has also prevented more radical conceptualisations which can lead to progressive change. Critical theory opens up such possibilities.

In this sense, the debate about universalism and relativism can also be regarded as a dialectic, and in seeking to hold the two together, critical theory can provide a framework within which the important critique of postmodernism can be maintained while at the same time allowing for a universalist (if deconstructed) humanist vision.

Within this paradigm, knowledge and action similarly cannot be separated, and the approach to practice which best incorporates such an integration is the dialogical method which has developed from the work of Freire (1972; see also McLaren and Leonard 1993; McLaren and Lankshear 1994). In this form of practice, the knowledge and wisdom of the worker are not privileged over the knowledge and wisdom of the 'client', and the relationship between the two is one of mutual education. Each learns from the other's experience, and as a result they can together engage in some form of action which may have been impossible for each in isolation. This requires a redefinition of the power relationship, and a reconstruction of the idea of 'professionalism'. It is consistent with Habermas's (1984, 1987) theory of 'communicative action', as Habermas—perhaps the foremost contemporary writer in critical theory—is concerned to retain some of the modernist notions of morality and justice, while freeing individuals to define their own realities and to act in order to improve their circumstances. The idea of achieving this through communication and the construction of discourse, and the suggestion that this represents a promising road to human liberation and can form the basis of human action, fits well with the aims and the practice of social work.

It is necessary for social workers to explore more rigorously, and in more detail, the philosophical grounding for their practice. As mentioned at the beginning of this chapter, the conventional frameworks have proved inadequate, and have not survived critiques from a range of theoretical and ideological perspectives. Social workers' interest in postmodernism is understandable, given the importance of the postmodernist critique, and the need to practise in an environment of increasing uncertainty and change. Postmodernism has a very important contribution to make to social work, but the contention of this chapter is that, by itself, it is insufficient, and would lead to a conservatising and inadequate form of practice. Critical theory, on the other hand, provides a paradigm within which the postmodernist critique can be largely incorporated, while at the same time fully legitimising social work's traditional commitments to universalist ideals of human rights and social justice. There can never be a complete explication of what such a social work might involve. Indeed, that would be a negation of the critical theory notion that it is only through some form of dialogical action that praxis can develop; to assume that conventional theoretical analysis alone can provide a basis for practice is to privilege the 'expert' knowledge of the practitioner or the academic, and hence to devalue the wisdom and knowledge of those with whom social workers work on a daily basis. Practice that is about genuine empowerment can never be certain of where it is heading, but—contrary to the views of some postmodernists—it can, and indeed must, proceed in a way that takes account of universal value, moral and ethical principles, even if the way in which these are defined and operationalised will vary over time and across cultural settings.

REFERENCES

Bauman, Z. (1993) *Postmodern Ethics*, Blackwell, Oxford
Carroll, J. (1993) *Humanism: The Wreck of Western Culture*, Fontana, London

Doyal, L. and Gough, I. (1991) *A Theory of Human Need*, Macmillan, London

Galtung, J. (1994) *Human Rights in Another Key*, Polity Press, Cambridge

——(1996) 'On the Social Costs of Modernization: Social Disintegration, Atomie/Anomie and Social Development', in C. de Alcántra (ed.), *Social Futures, Global Visions*, Blackwell, Oxford, pp. 165–99

Habermas, J. (1984) *The Theory of Communicative Action—Volume 1: Reason and the Rationalization of Society*, (trans. T. McCarthy), Beacon Press, Boston

——(1987) *The Theory of Communicative Action—Volume 2: Lifeworld and System: A Critique of Functionalist Reason* (trans. T. McCarthy), Beacon Press, Boston

Ife, J. (1997) *Rethinking Social Work: Towards Critical Practice*, Longman, Melbourne

Leonard, P. (1997) *Postmodern Welfare: Reconstructing an Emancipatory Project*, Sage, London

McLaren, P. and Lankshear, C. (eds) (1994) *Politics of Liberation: Paths from Freire*, Routledge, London

McLaren, P. and Leonard, P. (eds) (1993) *Paulo Freire: A Critical Encounter*, Routledge, London

Plumwood, V. (1993) *Feminism and the Mastery of Nature*, Routledge, London

Ray, L. (1993) *Rethinking Critical Theory: Emancipation in the Age of Global Social Movements*, Sage, London

Rosenau, P. (1992) *Post-modernism and the Social Sciences*, Princeton University Press, Princeton

Tönnies, F. (1955) *Community and Association* (trans. Loomis), Routledge, London

15 Emancipatory social work for a postmodern age
Jan Fook and Bob Pease

How have the chapters in this book developed possibilities for social work practice from a postmodern critical perspective, and what further questions need to be explored? In this final chapter, we will integrate the main themes and issues raised in the book: rethinking modernist social work concepts, reconstructing our educational practice and addressing the political dilemmas and possibilities. We conclude by engaging with some of the major criticisms directed at postmodern critical theory and its relevance to emancipatory social work.

RETHINKING MODERNIST SOCIAL WORK CONCEPTS

Most chapters are premised on the notion that traditional modernist notions are inadequate in representing practice experience, and have therefore begun with an analysis of existing social work theories or practices. The critique has been developed to formulate principles from which new ways of thinking and practice may be forged. In this section, we will outline some of these major principles.

1 *Reconceptualising the links between theory, practice and research.* The oppositional characterisation of theory and practice in social work, and the limitations of this conceptualisation in understanding and developing social work experience, comprise a major theme for both of us. We both experienced a disquiet about the split ways in which theory and practice were taught—Bob felt disquiet over the split between radical theory and practice; Jan was concerned by the clash between the espoused theory and the 'lived' experience

of radicalism. The theory/practice split was also a major issue for Peter Camilleri.

A postmodern view, which recognises that the dichotomisation of theory and practice is a modernist construct, allows for a more relevant conceptualisation of experience, so that theory is seen as a way of constructing meaning from concrete experience. Social work practice theory thus arises out of concrete and direct experience, and is developed in context; it must therefore be understood in relation to that context. Jan Fook's chapter on critical reflection illustrates how research can be linked with theorising practice experience, so that theory, practice and research are interconnected. Perhaps a way forward is to create a new language which does not carry such dichotomous connotations. We could speak about meaning, action and investigation, or about experience as an holistic phenomenon.

2 *Rethinking the organisational context of social work.* Postmodern critical theory criticises the meta-narratives of organisational efficiency and hierarchy as the dominant discourse of organisational life. Gary Hough suggests that clusters, networks, alliances and flat, flexible structures will displace the bureaucratic form of organisation as we move into the next century. Such developments allow for the construction of counter-discursive interventions by social workers and service users against the bureaucratic discourse and support for attempts to create alternative organisational forms.

3 *Rethinking the concept of power.* The modernist concept of power, and the associated identity categorisation, is questioned by Karen Healy, Karen Crinall and Stephen Parker et al. for its potentially disempowering effects. By conceptualising power as a commodity, identities are forced into 'powerful/powerless' or 'victim/helper' dualisms which do not do justice to either multiple diverse experiences, or the agency inherent in the choice (in the case of some young women) to follow a non-mainstream pathway. According to Karen Crinall, some homeless young women may construct their identities as a form of survival in difficult circumstances, rather than define themselves in deference to mainstream lifestyles. Karen Healy suggests that we need to understand and construct power by negotiating power relations in each context. In this way, the emphasis is on the fluid and changing processes of power. Karen Crinall suggests that we need to recognise and reframe 'victimhood' as resistance and survival against remarkable odds. Stephen Parker et al. adapt Minow's (1985) concept of 'the dilemma of difference' to reformulate

empowerment from a postmodern perspective. All three approaches open up new avenues for reconstructing power relations in society.

4 *Affirming the importance of agency*. The issue of agency is crucial to the emancipatory project. For Bob Pease, a postmodern critical perspective opens up new forms of resistance to dominant forms of masculinity. By exploring the subjectivities and practices of profeminist men, he argues that the postmodern concept of the decentred subject has greater critical potential for provoking inner change in men than the humanist notion of an innate self. He demonstrates how the contradictions in patriarchal discourses enables men, as well as women, to construct (pro)feminist subjectivities committed to egalitarian gender relations.

5 *Acknowledging diversity, difference and multiple subjectivities*. Many of the chapters have argued that recognising difference, diversity and multiple perspectives is empowering, and is indeed a necessity if codes and principles of practice are to be relevant to the many different groups of people with whom social workers associate. Linda Briskman and Carolyn Noble stress that we must engage in an ongoing project of interaction and dialogue to reformulate practices and codes which are relevant to particular groups or constituencies, in particular contexts. Lee FitzRoy acknowledges the political dilemmas, however, which are inherent in such a position. The political struggle risks becoming diluted if the focus is directed towards difference and experiences which do not necessarily bear out the collective argument. The risk is that the collective struggle disintegrates into a new type of individualism. How is difference to be celebrated, when collective solutions are sought at a structural level?

Perhaps an answer lies in recognising that a process of dialogue and partnership, which also respectfully acknowledges difference, may be an effective pathway to discovering commonality. Perhaps the critical postmodern pathway is one of process and dialogue, and in this process relationships are formed which encourage diverse people to act together. Hearing, recognising and valuing difference may be the first step towards inspiring people to act collectively.

RECONSTRUCTING EDUCATIONAL PRACTICE

Because of the uncertainties and the unfinished nature of postmodern thinking and acting, the education of social work students becomes potentially more difficult. The process of postmodern critical analysis necessarily involves a critical deconstruction of received ways of thinking. This process can be unsettling for many students, particularly when the work for which they will be employed will require decisive and effective action, often in situations which are unpredictable and beyond their control. The chapters in this book which deal with educational aspects begin from a position of deconstructing present thinking, but then continue to develop alternative approaches based on postmodern critical theorising. Helen Jessup and Steve Rogerson do this in relation to interpersonal communication theory and practice, and Lister Bainbridge in relation to mental health. Jan Fook's chapter articulates a process whereby students and practitioners can uncover or deconstruct their own approaches to practice, thereby laying a foundation for reconstructing their practice theory in ways more amenable to the emancipatory project. A challenge for social work education from a postmodern critical perspective is to foster in students the confidence to enter new situations prepared for dialogue and uncertainty, and with the creative tools to resist, challenge and reconstruct processes which will be more affirming for all parties. We hope that the process of critical reflection, throughout the chapters in this book, will help social work students and practitioners to begin this endeavour.

REASSESSING THE POLITICAL POSSIBILITIES

Jim Ife has raised serious concerns about the relevance and applicability of postmodern theorising to critical social work. He believes that critical social work's commitment to counter-oppressive practice may be undermined and weakened by the postmodern rejection of the meta-narrative. He is also concerned that the postmodern scepticism of universal principles may be used to justify the oppression of minorities.

We share these concerns, and we distance ourselves from those expressions of postmodernism that reject a commitment to social justice. We believe, however, that these issues are best addressed by linking progressive postmodern thinking with critical perspectives, to formulate a postmodern critical approach, transforming both postmodern theory and critical theory in the process. Jim differs from us in that he argues that critical theory *per se* can encompass what is useful and progressive in postmodernism. Rather than incorporating the postmodern critique within critical theory, as Jim advocates, we believe that many of the modernist premises of critical theory need to be rethought in light of the postmodern critique.

We find Hirschmann's (1992) distinction between postmodern feminism and feminist postmodernism useful in this regard. She agrees with those who argue that the tenets of postmodern theory make the concept of an emancipatory feminism impossible, but maintains—we think correctly—that there can be a postmodern feminism that uses deconstruction and other postmodern methods to deconstruct patriarchy and allow the marginalised voices to be heard. It is for this reason that we use postmodern as an adjective instead of postmodernism as a noun throughout this book.

We believe that one of the difficulties in accepting postmodern thinking lies in the modernist assumption that theoretical positions are mutually exclusive, implying that one can have allegiance to only one at a time. It is our contention that postmodern thinking does not attempt to posit one underlying causal explanation for phenomena. Thus there is no logical reason why aspects of postmodern thinking cannot sit easily with other causal theories, since it does not seek to *replace* other explanations, but rather to make observations about our process of *deriving* explanations.

In this sense, we have ongoing questions about how postmodern critical thinking can be helpful in specific concrete situations, rather than about whether it is should replace all existing theories. One of the difficulties we have found in introducing a postmodern critical perspective to students is that they sometimes feel they have to give up all past ways of thinking in order to embrace the new. We invite them to consider the idea that a postmodern perspective offers a *new way of thinking about thinking*, rather than trying to *replace the content of their old ways of thinking*. This emphasis on process is evident in Mary Lane's chapter, where she stresses the importance of openness and uncertainty, responsiveness to context, resistance to imposed agendas and values and rejection of arrogant professionalism which privileges expert knowledge over lived experience.

We also acknowledge that there is a need to further refine the political agenda of a postmodern approach. Partly because postmodern thinking allows a refocusing on the personal and individual, many progressive thinkers mistake this for an *apolitical* agenda. Modernist conceptions of power have determinedly located political struggles at the structural level, so that power tends to be associated only with collective, 'objective' struggles.

We believe that political struggles must take place on all different levels, since this is how life is experienced. We believe that it is important to change the modernist dichotomy that separates the individual from the social so that we are able to locate ourselves, reflexively, into a holistic contextual picture. From our point of view, postmodern critical thinking is important for emancipatory practice because it puts the individual back in the picture, while at the same time contributing to a reconstruction of the social. In the process of transforming ourselves, we contribute to social transformation through prefiguring alternative subjectivities and practices. The choices today of practitioners, educators, students and service users will form the basis of the collective politics of the future. We hope that this book contributes both to the transformation of individual lives and to the reconstruction of the emancipatory collective project.

REFERENCE

Hirschmann, N. (1992) *Rethinking Obligation: A Feminist Method for Political Theory*, Cornell University Press, Ithaca

Index